UNLOCKED

UNLOCKED

A Family Emerging from the Shadows of Autism

Susan Levin

Afterword by Donna Gates

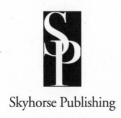

Skyhorse Publishing

All rights reserved. No part of this book may be reproduced in any manner without the express written consent of the publisher, except in the case of brief excerpts in critical reviews or articles. All inquiries should be addressed to Skyhorse Publishing, 307 West 36th Street, 11th Floor, New York, NY 10018.

Skyhorse Publishing books may be purchased in bulk at special discounts for sales promotion, corporate gifts, fund-raising, or educational purposes. Special editions can also be created to specifications. For details, contact the Special Sales Department, Skyhorse Publishing, 307 West 36th Street, 11th Floor, New York, NY 10018 or info@skyhorsepublishing.com.

Skyhorse® and Skyhorse Publishing® are registered trademarks of Skyhorse Publishing, Inc.®, a Delaware corporation.

The Son-Rise Program® and the Option Process® are registered trademarks of Barry Neil Kaufman and Susan Marie Kaufman. Autism Treatment Center of America® is a registered trademark of The Option Institute and Fellowship.

Visit our website at www.skyhorsepublishing.com.

10 9 8 7 6 5 4 3 2 1

Library of Congress Cataloging-in-Publication Data is available on file.

Cover design by Owen Corrigan

Print ISBN: 978-1-63220-719-7
Ebook ISBN: 978-1-63220-804-0

Printed in the United States of America

This book is dedicated to all parents, but especially my own.
And, of course, to Sean.

Contents

Introduction
A Practical Hope

I *hung up the phone from a conversation with a friend and walked into the living room. I saw my infant daughter, Alina, asleep in her bassinet, and smiled. But wait a minute—where was Ben, my three-year-old? Hadn't he been with Alina in the living room just moments before? How long had I been on the phone?*

"Ben?" I called out hopefully. No answer. I walked through the first floor, searching. My heart began to pound. "BenBen? BenBen? Ben, honey, where are you, sweetheart?" I could hear the anxiety in my voice. I knew my hollering was useless; Ben never answered me, even when he was right in front of me. But where could he be?

I ran upstairs, looked in his room, then in ours, and then in the bathrooms. He was nowhere to be found. I ran downstairs again, through the kitchen. I ran into the living room to check on Alina, who was still asleep, blissfully unaware of her mother's hysteria. I ran outside, into the front yard. "BENJAMIN? WHERE ARE YOU? BENBEN? ANSWER MOMMY!"

By now I was crying, tears streaming down my face. I was in a state of utter terror, my mind filled with horrible visions of children stolen away from right under their parents' noses, terrible images of kidnappers and perpetrators and everything I'd ever seen on television. I raced around to the back of the house. He wasn't there. I ran back inside, called the po-

lice, and then called my husband. I ran out into the front yard again. I screamed Ben's name over and over again. No one came. I couldn't breathe. I felt as if my world were ending.

Then I saw him. He was in the next-door neighbor's yard, no more than a few hundred feet away. He had sneaked through the fence and was playing on their slide. He had been there the whole time, deaf to my screams, insensible to my hysterical, sobbing pleas, oblivious to all but himself and his own experience. He went up and down the slide, ignoring me, never registering my voice, my terror, or my pain. All of that was irrelevant. He was on his slide.

My relief was intense, but so, too, was my rage. How could he have put me through that? Why didn't he respond to my cries? Didn't he care that his own mother was in pain? How could he ignore me that way? Then I began to berate myself. How could I have let him get outside? What if he had really been taken from me? What kind of mother was I?

It took me years to discover that I was asking the wrong questions. Ben's behavior wasn't about *me*. He wasn't ignoring *me*. The problem was not in *me*. It took our family several more years of pain, turmoil, and confusion to finally understand: Ben had autism.

***

On March 27, 2014, the Centers for Disease Control (CDC) announced new statistics on autism. According to their research, autism now affects one in sixty-eight children, and one in forty-two boys. That means virtually every grade in every elementary school has at least one child with autism.[1]

In the 1970s, only 1 in 10,000 children had an autism diagnosis. In the 1980s, many argue in relation to the addition of new, compulsory

---

1   *USA Today,* March 28, 2014, "Autism rates soar, now affects 1 in 68 children."

vaccines, this figure rose to 1 in every 2,500.[2] As of February 2007, the CDC put the incidence of autism at 1 in 150 children and 1 out of 90 boys.[3] The CDC has used the same method to determine autism prevalence every two years since 2000 and showed a 120 percent increase in autism rates between 2000 and 2010.[4] Autism is an epidemic of apocalyptic proportions, which attacks the very heart of our society: families and our children's capacity to establish and sustain relationships with others.

In addition to the epidemic of autism, another epidemic abounds today—one of hopelessness and resignation on the part of medical professionals, parents, and other caregivers. The collective national belief is that *autism cannot be cured.* The American Academy of Pediatrics states on its website, on a page titled, "Autism Facts," that "although there is no cure, autism is treatable." An October 23, 2006, online article titled, "Autism: An Incurable Developmental Disability,"[5] states, "Developmental disability is an expression employed to refer to serious life long impairment that substantially reduces one or more of one's life functions. . . . One of such disabilities is Autism."

In an article published in *The New York Times Magazine* on July 31, 2014, journalist Ruth Padawer wrote the following:

> Autism is considered a lifelong developmental disorder, but its diagnosis is based on a constellation of behavioral symptoms—social difficulties, fixated interests, obsessive or repetitive actions and unusually intense or dulled reactions to sensory stimulation—because no reliable

2   *NewsWithViews.com,* November 13, 2007, Dr. Carolyn Dean and Melissa Meininger, "Autism Can Be Treated"
3   Ibid., Dean and Meisinger.
4   Carolyn Klein online article, "Autism Is Curable"
5   From *ArticlesFactory,* http://www.articlesfactory.com/articles/health/autism-an-incurable-developmental-disability.html.

bio-markers exist. Though the symptoms of autism frequently become less severe by adulthood, the consensus has always been that its core symptoms remain. Most doctors have long dismissed as wishful thinking the idea that someone can recover from autism. Supposed cures have been promoted on the Internet—vitamin shots, nutritional supplements, detoxifiers, special diets, pressurized rooms filled with pure oxygen and even chelation, the potentially dangerous removal of heavy metals from the body. But no evidence indicates that any of them can alleviate any of the core symptoms of autism, let alone eradicate it.

To date, our society has taught us to believe that autism is a lifelong and irreversible condition, with no hope for cure. This book is a challenge to that belief and an invitation to parents of children on the autism spectrum to believe that *their children can heal.*

Autism first entered our life as a curse, when our toddler, Ben, displayed undiagnosed, aberrant behavior, and then, later, when Ben received an autism diagnosis, we felt ourselves to be victims of what we believed to be a chronic developmental disorder. But as we desperately sought out, discovered, and implemented a number of different interventions, we learned that what we had been told—that autism was irreversible—was simply not true. With that new understanding and our newborn commitment to curing Ben of autism, we set out on a path that strengthened us, transformed us, and taught us how to truly and unconditionally love our children—and ourselves.

Could we believe in our child's potential? It was a hard question. Hope was a frightening prospect. So many warned against the dangers of false hope.

I am a strong person. I am a Harvard College graduate, I was a lawyer in Boston, and, if you met me, you would probably say that I present as a stable and intelligent person. But this road, the one I chose and that I describe in this book, is tough. Even for strong people.

I wrote this book because when our son was diagnosed with autism, I hit an emotional low like I had never known before. I was desperate and terribly overwhelmed. Most articles I read and most professionals with whom my husband and I consulted, said the same thing: autism was a lifelong sentence, and the most we could hope for was managed care. But those prospects were intolerable, and I set off on a quest to recover my son, whom I loved more than anything in my life.

What happened? I found many things that worked. I found many things that didn't work. But I kept on, and ultimately, I came to understand the roots of my son's autism and discover the methods by which we could address and improve his condition. It took us over six years, thousands of dollars, and many tough days. Thousands of hard moments. We made choices others called "sacrifices." People called us noble and "incredible parents." But we didn't do any of it to be noble. I don't think we're more incredible than anyone else. We just love our children. We didn't feel we had a choice, because we wanted so badly for our son to get well.

But it's a tough path.

Ben is now twelve years old. He has come a long way in the six years since he received his diagnosis. He is not cured of challenges, but he has shed many of his autistic symptoms. Through this journey, Ben has become an expressive, compassionate, and—most significantly—a connected young boy.

In this book, I use the phrase "autism recovery," by which I mean having both the desire and the capacity to connect meaningfully with others. Autism is a spectrum, and many people—diagnosed or not—fall somewhere on its continuum. Ben may never be "normal," and he may always be quirky, for lack of a better term. But he has, at this point, traveled far enough along a path of emergence, which began at total, deliberate disconnection and isolation, that he is now, most of the time, in a state of total, deliberate *connection* and meaningfully relating to other people. It's a great start.

Ben is not the only child who is journeying out of autism through the various interventions we implemented. Many families around the world, hit with this epidemic disorder, are healing their children through these means. We believe that most children with autism suffer from malfunctioning digestive systems and compromised immune and detoxification systems, which together produce impaired neural functioning. Many of these children work with professional therapists and caregivers who are unable to meet these children on their own terms and thus miss the opportunity to build a bridge into their autistic world—a bridge across which the children can eventually emerge into a world of healthy relations with others. Finally, many parents are unable—whether from fear or from lack of information—to discover the bridge across the chasm of disconnection, which can connect them to the children and create permanent healing. These parents need support and education.

Through the path we walked, however, we have made great headway in connecting with our son. Over the past six years, Ben emerged from autism, and we literally "got to know him"—years later than most parents begin to get to know their children. While Ben was still under the spell of autism, what we knew of him was mostly his autistic symptoms, many of which were very hard to live with and hard to accept. But as Ben emerged from autism, we began to find out who he was on the inside.

And who is Ben? Ben is a prolific story writer and storyteller. Ben's mind is sharp and fast. Ben is deeply compassionate and eager to please others. Ben loves fiercely. Ben is very funny—he's a punster! Ben loves reading. Ben's favorite sport is basketball, but he considers himself "an indoor boy" more than a sporty one. Ben loves riding his bike. Ben loves girls. Ben's favorite person in the world is his sister. Ben feels his Judaism deeply and is excited for his *bar mitzvah*, which will happen in two years. Ben loves Harry Potter. He has written seven children's books and is currently writing his eighth. He hopes to publish them on Amazon this year.

Ben has so many amazing qualities.

We had no idea.

Of course, all children reveal more of themselves as they develop. We constantly learn more about our other child, our daughter, Alina: who she is, what she loves, what she fears, and what she dreams. But when you have a child whose soul and character are hidden from you because of autism, the experience of finally getting to know them is different. It's unique and overwhelming at times. It has touched and healed our hearts. If your child does not have autism, you may not be able to understand the miracle of discovering your child when they emerge. But if your child has autism, I promise you: it is worth everything to try for recovery.

I wrote this book because I want to share Ben's story, for the hope it offers other families. He has come so far in six years that we have every reason to believe he could ultimately make a full recovery. Ben is, at this point, despite his progress, neither "cured" nor "neurotypical." He still has speech problems, his internal systems are not totally healthy, and he still suffers from distractibility and, at times, rigidity.

But he no longer appears to meet the profile of a child with autism. He is passionately interested in others, especially in his peers at school and at our temple. He is responsive, quick, and compassionate. He includes others in his activities. When members of his family are away, he misses them and says so. He reflects upon his errors, both academic and behavioral, and tries to correct them. When he knows I don't have time for him, he lets go, often graciously. He constantly expresses his desires, his thoughts, his feelings, and his inner life in a way that is not only *not* autistic, but that is, in fact, remarkable for an eleven-year-old. When his grandfather went into a coma earlier this year, Ben called him and said, "I'm sad you're dying, because I love you and miss you. I'm sad that I will never hear your voice again." At the funeral, Ben said to his grandmother, "This must be terribly hard for you," and hugged her tight.

If this is as far as we get, I'll take it. But I don't think Ben's progress will end here. He is motivated to grow and change. He tells us he wants to go to college, get married, have a family, and develop a career.

I wrote this book because I want every parent whose child receives an autism diagnosis to know that *there is hope*. Every child on the autism spectrum is different, even if they receive the same diagnosis, and there are no guarantees. But for the vast majority of children on the spectrum, we believe there is hope for major progress, if not total recovery, through the approaches we have explored and embraced, many of which I describe in this book. I wrote this book, because I want to share the lessons we have learned along the way, so other parents might not have to take as many years as we did to learn them.

Many people still don't believe recovery from autism is possible, but I know it is because of our experience with Ben. In this book, I offer not a methodology, but rather the experience of one family—an experience that we hope and believe to be transferrable, as the principles underlying our son's transformation apply to some extent to all children on the autism spectrum. I hope parents and caregivers reading this book will find hope that they, too, can discover their children, as we have discovered—and continue to discover—ours.

As Ben's mother on this journey, I also played the roles of nutritionist, clinician, doctor, teacher, therapist, scientist, special education practitioner, and private eye. I read, researched, pondered, experimented, and spent years in community with others on this path. I sought new information about healing, uncovered rational explanations for autistic behaviors, and ultimately found novel ways to help my son. If you talk to any parents who have chosen to attempt recovery for their child with autism, you will likely find they have worn many hats as well.

In the interest of authenticity and to encourage those parents who may feel as I did, it is important for me to note at the outset that most of the time with Ben, both before and after autism, *I believed that I was not doing a good enough job.* In my mind, I wasn't smart enough, organized enough, loving enough, creative enough, or rich enough. I didn't do a good enough job implementing the diets, the therapies, or the instructions of our trainers. I felt like a phony when people called me a great mom, because I felt wholly inadequate. Maybe it's just maternal psychology, but somehow mothers—even the strongest of us—usually don't see our own value. I know I didn't. Frankly, if I were reading a book about some mother who had done the things I have done, I would never have thought myself capable of such things.

I am not the "warrior-mother" type. I grew up in the DC area, an over-privileged young woman, who was blessed to receive a great education, find good work, and marry a wonderful man. I was much more comfortable reading a book or spending time with friends than playing with my own children. I knew with absolute certainty that home-schooling mothers were mentally ill, and school teachers only slightly less so. I was a different species. I wasn't into children. Also, despite an unexpected primal passion I felt when my son was born and then later when my daughter arrived, I had absolutely no confidence in my parenting abilities. I was actually terrified of being a mother.

But when it came to Ben's recovery, it turned out that none of my insecurities mattered. I had what it took, which was a willingness to go to any lengths to help Ben and to keep going when I didn't want to. (By the way, I don't think even my willingness was noble. It was borne of my wants. *I wanted* to know and connect with my son, and *I wanted* a decent life for my family, including myself.) Sometimes, I didn't even feel that I loved my son. I actually felt at times that I hated him, because his autism was so terrifying to me. But in the end, love beat out fear, and I stayed the course.

I hope this book will inspire other parents to believe in their children's potential for recovery. Children may represent the world's tomorrow, but I want my relationship with my child to be meaningful today. Like love, hope is only meaningful if it is practical. It must be accompanied by action. But with love, hope, and persistent action, there is no such thing as false hope for *any* child suffering from autism. Ben is a testament to that fact.

PART I:

A PATH
NOT CHOSEN

Chapter 1
Our "Perfect Baby"

I sat on the toilet screaming, my hip bones crushed, as though in a vise. I dropped to my knees, swayed back and forth, and tried to remember the lessons from our one and only natural-childbirth class. My mind was a blank. I waddled to the bathroom window, clutching my heaving belly. I looked out the window onto the driveway below. "Where are you, motherfucker!" I hollered to my absent husband, consumed by pain and terror.

It didn't make sense. The baby wasn't due for another five weeks. My water hadn't broken; there had been just a small trickle that morning. What was going on? And where was Sean? He should have been home by now!

The contraction subsided, and I hobbled into the walk-in closet next door. "I need a shirt for the hospital," I remembered. "They said to pack a bag!" I searched frantically for a shirt to pack. Two questions suddenly invaded my mind. First, "Is the baby dying?" Then, "Am I dying?" These thoughts were intolerable, and I shut them out of my mind at once. I began to pray fervently for God to help me survive this ordeal. Another contraction hit, and I fell to the floor, onto my back. The hardwood floor was no friend to me, as I lay there in back labor, agony ripping through my body.

Suddenly, I heard the front door open and Sean running up the stairs. He heard my screams, saw me, and instantly understood. He dialed 911 and yelled into the phone: "Sir, my wife's having a baby!" Suddenly I screamed: the baby had crowned; I reached down with my hand and felt his tiny, hairy head. Sean yelled again into the phone, "The head is out! The head is out!" The paramedic replied, clearly reading from some laminated card, "Sir, that's Step Nine! We're only on Step Two!" Ten seconds more, and another contraction. I screamed, pushed, and my son, my Benjamin, flew out of me, landing on the floor. He was blue and purple, but thankfully he cried immediately, pulling air into his tiny lungs.

My son had been born, the pain had ended, and our parenting journey had begun.

My son, Ben, arrived five weeks early, and weighed three pounds and twelve ounces at birth. I always believed he came early because he was so eager to get here. He had jaundice and lay in an incubator under ultraviolet light for his first few days. I stayed with him in the NICU for seventeen days, until he maintained his weight and temperature, and we were allowed to go home.

We survived our first night. In other words, when we woke up and Ben was still alive, we were happy, as are all new parents.

Despite a difficult pregnancy and an indescribable delivery, we were one of the happiest couples on earth when Ben was born. We had been through several years of fertility treatments in order to conceive Ben and had prayed for years to have a child of our own. I was an excited new mom, making my homemade baby food, considering and then quickly dispensing with the idea of cloth diapers, and inviting thrilled friends and family to come and meet Ben. We lived in a beautiful home, my husband's job was stable, and life felt exciting and wonderful, though scary in the newness of it all.

Ben was a happy infant. Unfortunately, he could barely nurse, because his mouth was too small to latch, but once he started eating, he gained weight well and thrived physically. He had all of the usual vaccinations, despite his low birth weight. He smiled all the time. Sean and I were both rather afraid of our new arrival, who looked more like a kitten—or E.T.—than like any newborn we'd ever seen. But I had many happy days during Ben's infancy. I did a lot of photography in those days. I'd bundle Ben up, and off we would drive to some old New England inn, cemetery, or other appealing location. I was so proud of my healthy, handsome, friendly baby boy with his huge, blue eyes, cherry lips, and beautiful smile.

Looking back at those early days, I don't remember him *not* responding to me. I just remember intense happiness, wonder, and amazement. My dream had finally come true. *I had a son.*

When my husband and I went out to eat, we thought we had the perfect baby. Ben would sit in his high chair or booster seat, calm, placid, and immobile. We would talk, laugh, and converse with each other for hours, and Ben wouldn't make a peep. I remember thinking, "His tush must have fallen asleep by now!" We had a lot of freedom, with our wonderfully behaved baby boy. Little did we realize that Ben was in a world of his own, far away, and disconnected from us. Ben liked to lie on his back at that age, staring upward at the ceiling. Other infants rolled, giggled, followed your pointing finger, and noticed other babies. But not Ben. He just laid on his back, smiling, in his faraway world.

I started noticing real differences in Ben's play style when he was about two years old. Other mothers, friends of mine, would come over for playdates or group lunches, and I could see Ben was different from the other toddlers. The other children were beginning to interact with one another and were playing with the toys and blocks lying everywhere around them. Ben, however, continued his infantile behavior of lying on his back, smiling, seemingly unaware of the toys and children around him.

When Ben was two and a half, I brought in Early Intervention, who diagnosed Ben with a seventeen-month *global delay*, meaning that his speech and both his gross and fine-motor skills were very behind for his age. At their recommendation, we began physical, occupational, and speech therapy. He made no noticeable improvement in any area, however. When Ben was three years old, I enrolled him in a special-needs preschool near our home. They gave him ABA (Applied Behavioral Analysis), as well as other standard therapies. Again, we saw no changes behaviorally. He continued to smile constantly, and he also continued to ignore people and things around him, except for foods he loved, which were typically starchy, cheesy, and meaty foods like mac and cheese, milk, and hot dogs.

As Ben got a bit older, his behavior worsened. He became rigid, controlling, prone to tantrums, and even more of a picky eater, seemingly addicted to certain foods and eating them in large quantities. He rarely, if ever, looked in our eyes.

His language was repetitive. Ben had a pronounced auditory-processing delay: he would sometimes answer a question minutes after the question was asked, or sometimes not at all. He spent hours playing the same repetitive games and excluding the world around him.

Ben also suffered from anxiety. If we went near a playground with children on it, even a single child, Ben panicked, began to shake and cry, and showed a primal compulsion to flee.

Ben exhibited a profound lack of communication with others. He used words—though they were unintelligible to most people—but he rarely chose to use them to communicate. We had no conversation "loops"; that is, I say something, you respond, and that equals one loop. I never knew what he was thinking or feeling, only the obvious:

if he grinned, he was happy; if he cried, he was either sad or distressed. But Ben did not directly communicate with us. He seemed to have no interest in others.

He did, however, show a definite affection for his little sister, Alina, who is two years younger than he is. But he never said, "I love you, Mommy," or "I love you, Daddy." If we tried to hug him, Ben went limp in our arms.

In school or at playdates, Ben seemed unaware of other children or adults. Ben did not actually play with other children but rather played *by himself in the presence of other children*, what child development specialists call "parallel play." At his preschool, Ben had one "friend," another boy with autism. In truth, though they seemed to enjoy each other's company, they didn't actually play *together*. When I visited Ben's preschool class one day, Ben was in his own world, neither talking to the other children nor engaging in activities with them.

Ben had a decided need for strong sensory stimulation that started very early, probably because his brain was not sending enough of a sensory punch to his limbs. When Ben started to crawl, he military crawled at light speed. His military crawl had me *running* after him. He clearly liked the feeling of moving, and of moving fast.

Additionally, when Ben was between the ages of three and five years old, he often bolted from places, running and running, sometimes without me realizing he had fled the scene. One time, for example, we were at a friend's house, and Ben was in another room playing with trains. Without my knowing it, he slipped outside and took off down the block. I didn't realize he was gone until many minutes later (I'll never know how many), and in a total panic, I ran down the street, eventually driving in my minivan, shouting out his name over and over again. It turned out, a kind family had seen my little toddler walking alone down the street and had coerced him inside with the promise of ice cream, which he was very much enjoying when I pulled up in the minivan. I remember realizing, "Oh my God, he will go with anyone who offers him ice cream!"

Then there was the time Ben sneaked off into the woods behind our old house, running down a trail for a long while on his own, and we had to call the police to come find him. At that time, they wanted us to put a GPS bracelet on his ankle. I declined.*

There are quite a few more examples of Ben's cutting and bolting, a behavior in which many children on the spectrum engage. On a purely sensory level, Ben seemed to love the feeling of the wind pushing against him, of flying, and of being in motion. But for me, the most striking aspect of that behavior was the total, apparent lack of awareness of the impact of his disappearances on others (*i.e.*, *me*). I also observed, at those times, an absence of appropriate fear at being away from his caregivers and alone in a strange environment. These are symptoms of autism to me—a psychological or neurological disconnect from his impact on others, or their impact on him.

Then there were the tantrums.

When Ben lived in autism, we lived as prisoners to Ben's daily temper tantrums. Our entire world revolved around avoiding Ben's tantrums. If he lost a favorite toy, my husband would drive miles and go to possibly multiple toy stores to retrieve or replace the toy rather than face Ben's massive histrionics. When we drove to or from anywhere, Ben had a tantrum. If we were on the highway and he wanted the back roads, he cried, screamed, and raged as if his life were at stake. If we were on the back roads, and he wanted the highway, I'd drive twenty minutes out of the way just to find a highway. If I refused to comply with his wishes, Ben would punish me with ten, twenty, thirty, forty,

---

* Ben actually communicated *his* experience of this event to me years later, after he emerged from autism. (See blog entry November 11, 2013.)

or more minutes of screaming and crying. It just wasn't worth the tantrum that would ensue if Ben didn't get his way, so I always gave in.

I was exhausted all the time and felt a deep sense of inadequacy as a mother. I simply couldn't understand him. I felt completely unable to comfort my child, and it hurt that he did not seem to desire my help. He seemed, in fact, barely aware of me as a person, much less as his mother. Much less as someone he *loved*.

Ben was obsessive to the point of frenzy. I remember one summer when Ben, Alina, and I drove every day to Camp Triumph, a special-needs camp Ben attended when he was five. Every day, as we drove, Ben needed to hear a particular song. I don't remember the actual name of the song, but we called it the "Uggi Song." It was a cute, syncopated piece from a children's CD we got from the Handwriting Without Tears company. Ben adored it. Relentlessly, every morning, we had to hear that song over and over and over again. After camp, Ben would play it on the computer, and he would ride his tricycle around the kitchen, merrily listening to the same song. Always, Ben sought sameness, predictability, and control.

Ben repeatedly asked the same question, for example, as often as twenty or thirty times a day. I thought he was trying to be difficult; I couldn't understand how he possibly could not know the answer after the one hundredth time I had given it. Later, I learned that Ben's world felt totally unpredictable and uncertain, and by asking the same question repeatedly—with a guarantee that he would receive the same answer—he created a sense of predictability, certainty, and control for himself. How ingenious! As I came to understand my child's strategies and possible intentions, I became able to let go of the judgments and fears my lack of understanding had instilled in me. But all of that understanding came much later, and in our early years, when Ben asked questions like that, I became instantly infuriated and upset.

We couldn't do "normal" family activities. Every event turned into an emotional catastrophe. If we went to a restaurant (which was rare), Ben completely checked out, and often put his head in my lap under the table to avoid any contact with people. Today, I believe he was over-stimulated and unable to process the multitude of sensations and feelings coming at him. So he took care of himself by checking out in order to avoid further stimulation. But at the time, I just felt embarrassed and even angry at Ben for behaving so "oddly" and for being so different from other children. I was angry at myself as well, because, again, I felt incompetent as a mother. Why was my kid so weird? It had to be my fault. After all, he was my child, and I was his mother.

One of my worst memories was a birthday party Ben attended when he was four and in special-needs preschool. The party took place at an ice-cream parlor, and the children—a group of squealing four-year-olds—were served enormous bowls of vanilla ice cream. All around the table were smaller bowls filled with candies of all kinds, which the children were invited to put on top of their ice cream. Ben ignored the candy but ate almost his entire trough of ice cream. After the ice cream, all of the children gathered in the back of the room to play party games with the staff.

Ben, however, didn't seem to even see the other children or the party staff. Instead of joining in the games, he wandered the circumference of the room, his hands and face pressed upon the wallpaper, feeling its texture. I stood and watched him, tears in my eyes welling up almost unbearably. Usually in social situations, on the outside I tried to present myself as a charming, cheerful, and upbeat mom, pretending it didn't bother me that my son was totally in his own world, disconnected from every other human being in the room. But on the inside, I cried and felt sorry for our family, myself, and Ben.

We became isolated as a family. When Ben was an infant, my husband and I held large parties at our home. Ten, twenty, thirty, or more of our friends came for cookouts, holiday parties, and other get-togethers. But after Ben became a toddler, and his behavior became more erratic and even volatile, we stopped having people over. Our social life disappeared and with it, our sense of fun and connection with our community. Although we stayed in contact with the important members of our family and closest friends, most of the time we were too scared and embarrassed by Ben's behavior to venture out of our house.

Our isolation damaged us both emotionally and psychologically. My husband and I are both social people who enjoy community. But we assumed no one would understand what we were going through. I remember having conversations with friends of ours, parents of "normal" children, and feeling angry, envious, and self hating, because I blamed myself for Ben's problems. I remember thinking, "How can you be saying these things to me?" as they described their "difficult trip to Disney." Did they not understand that Disney World was off the table for us? Did they know how much I would give for a "difficult trip to Disney?" How much I would give even to have a single conversation with my son?

I experienced both self-pity and anger toward those I considered insensitive to our pain, parents of "normal" children who, from where I was sitting, didn't know how good they had it. I was angry, isolated, and lonely. I mourned the child I had envisioned, who was *not* the child in front of me.

At that point in our life, I was terrified for Ben's future and for ours. I felt angry at circumstances and at myself for not knowing how to make everything better. I experienced despondency, because I knew I didn't know how to help my son. I was also utterly exhausted—spiritually, emotionally, physically, and mentally.

Chapter 2
Diagnosis and Possibilities

*N*o one—family members, teachers, doctors, or other caregivers— ever suggested to us that Ben had autism. In fact, I remember thinking, some time before Ben received his diagnosis, "Thank God, at least we don't have *that*!"

Then, in October 2007, two and a half years after the Early Intervention assessment, a friend suggested I take Ben to a pediatric neuropsychologist in our town. This doctor tested Ben over a period of three days. A week later, we met with the doctor, and he told us Ben was most definitely on the autism spectrum. My first reaction was shock. Then tears. Then terror. Everyone knew autism was a lifelong disorder and couldn't be cured.

The doctor gave us little information or guidance as to where to go from there. He made a small diagram, indicating different approaches parents and caregivers typically implement to address the disorder, including behavioral therapy, nutrition, and the usual round of speech therapy, occupational therapy, and physical therapy. He remarked, toward the end of the conversation, "Ben's prognosis is good. He might go to college."

Both my husband and I are intellectuals with advanced degrees. Now a well-credentialed doctor was telling us that our son *might* go to college, and we were devastated. The world was spinning. Autism was not in my plan. We walked out of that doctor's office broken, demoralized, and filled with apprehension about our new life—as parents of a child with autism.

As soon as we recovered from the shock, we mobilized ourselves and started researching our options. We tried to find a strategy but found ourselves overwhelmed by the sheer number of interventions available. Ultimately, what unfolded from that point in October 2007 was a journey that became the focus of our lives. Through the discovery and implementation of three central paradigms of healing—namely, biomedical interventions, our Son-Rise Program (a child-driven, home-based, social-relational program), and comprehensive tools for self care as parents—our son, our family, and our spirits healed.

BIOMEDICAL INTERVENTIONS: AN OVERVIEW

The first paradigm we explored was biomedical intervention, which refers to the healing of the body, with special focus on digestion and the gastrointestinal tract, in order to heal the brain. During the first year after Ben received his diagnosis, I read books about children recovering through supplements and better nutrition, and I also learned about the DAN! ("Defeat Autism Now!") Protocol. DAN! was a movement of medical professionals and concerned parents and caregivers of children with autism.

DAN! was a project of the Autism Research Institute (ARI), which was founded in the 1960s by Dr. Bernard Rimland.*

---

* ARI was founded in 1967 by Bernard Rimland, PhD, a research psychologist. Rimland's book, *Infantile Autism: The Syndrome and Its Implications for a Neural Theory of Behavior*, was published in 1964. Rimland was the first to authoritatively challenge the prevailing theory of the time, the refrigerator-mother theory (that autism was caused by unloving mothers), by providing evidence that autism is a biological disorder. (From http://en.wikipedia.org/wiki/Autism_Research_Institute.) DAN! as a term is now obsolete; the current vernacular is biomedical interventions.

DAN! doctors were trained in the DAN! Protocol, an approach to autism treatment premised on the idea that autism is a biomedical disorder. Specifically, DAN! doctors felt that autism is a disorder caused by a combination of lowered immune response, external toxins from vaccines and other sources, and problems caused by certain foods, among other factors.

In an article called "Advice to Parents of Children with Autism,"* authors associated with ARI said this:

> Routine medical tests are usually performed by traditional pediatricians, but these exams rarely reveal underlying medical problems that are often associated with autism, such as gastrointestinal problems, nutritional and metabolic deficiencies, toxic metal burden, and immune dysfunction. Unfortunately, many physicians believe, though incorrectly, that the only useful medical treatments are psychiatric medications to reduce seizures and behavioral problems.
>
> The Autism Research Institute supports an integrative medical approach to treating individuals on the autism spectrum. This approaches often includes:
> - Nutritional supplements, including certain vitamins, minerals, amino acids, and essential fatty acids
> - Special diets totally free of gluten (from wheat, barley, rye, and possibly oats), free of dairy (milk, ice-cream, yogurt, etc.), and free of soy

---

* James B. Adams, Ph.D., Stephen M. Edelson, Ph.D., Temple Grandin, Ph.D., Bernard Rimland, Ph.D., Jane Johnson "Advice for Parents of Young Autistic Children" (2012, Revised), Autism Research Institute, http://www.autism.com/understanding_advice.

- Testing for hidden food allergies, and avoidance of allergenic foods
- Treatment of intestinal bacterial/yeast overgrowth
- Detoxification

The biomedical model appealed to me, as we had met with little support or information from our local pediatrician. So I found a DAN! doctor an hour from our home and, at his recommendation, put Ben cold turkey onto a gluten-free/casein-free diet. We quickly noticed radical shifts in Ben's disposition; he was calmer, seemed more aware of us, and was a little less spacey.

I continued to read articles about the biomedical approach to autism recovery. My head swam with information about yeast, enzymes, and something called "Leaky Gut Syndrome." Upon the advice of our new DAN! doctor, we began giving Ben weekly vitamin B12 shots and daily doses of various supplements, including fish oil, GABA, DMG, and numerous other foul-smelling and foul-tasting items. It was very difficult to get Ben to take these things, but we were committed. We were also hopeful, because Ben seemed to be connecting more.

But the changes were limited. At five years old, Ben needed more than just biomedical interventions to recover fully from autism. The articles I read about children with autism fully recovering through the DAN! protocol were mostly about toddlers. By five, Ben's brain had hardwired a lot of aberrant socialization patterns, and he needed more than just organic healing. He had a lot of unlearning to do.

We remained hopeful, but still scared. We had no one to talk to except doctors who were unsupportive of our biomedical interventions (the only thing we had found that had helped at all), teachers who seemed to have nothing to offer besides much-needed (but not curative) compassion and kindness, and therapists of various kinds (speech therapy, occupational therapy, hippotherapy) who offered no hope for actually curing Ben's autism.

We had no community. We knew almost no other parents with children on the spectrum and none at all who believed autism could be cured. We were overworked and stressed to the maximum. We fought constantly, even in front of the children, which we had sworn we would never do, venting our anxiety on each other. We didn't stop to think; there was no time. We continued to hunt for answers, solutions, anything that might help.

Every family facing autism faces an enormous array of interventions, and we were no different. Because of the epidemic numbers of children afflicted, autism has become a market of different diets, therapies, and practitioners, all touting their wares as the be-all, end-all cure. Navigating that market is overwhelming, regardless of your background or educational level. I again felt inadequate, and depression was a constant temptation. I prayed for guidance, but I felt lost.

And always, underneath, were our fears: Ben would never go to college. He would never have a family. He would never know intimacy, emotional fulfillment, or creative and fulfilling work. We were terrified, but we kept going, always looking. Always hoping.

PART II:

A LONG JOURNEY

Chapter 3
Emergence

*B*en sat on the floor, lining up his ABA-schedule cards. Never noticing what was on the card, he placed each one carefully in its own
spot, at the intersection of the wall and the floor. I watched him for a
few moments, then sat down a few yards away from him, and began to
line up my own set of ABA cards, one by one, each in its own spot, at
the intersection of the wall and the floor. I played in my mind, imagining a schedule for an ideal day for myself. I placed my first card: out
to breakfast with my husband. I placed the second card: off to Barnes
& Noble to pick up some books. I placed my third card: back home to
finish a project. On I went, peacefully placing my cards, all the while
aware of Ben's movements, his focus on his cards, and his seeming lack of
awareness that I was in the room.

Day after day, hour after hour, I joined him, placing cards one after
another, in endless lines, Ben consistently failing to show any interest in me
or acknowledge my presence in any way.

One day, as I was placing my cards, enjoying my imaginary schedule
for that day, Ben suddenly looked at me. He saw me. He did a double take,
and then he grinned. Utterly startled, I yelled, "Hi, Ben!" A moment later, I
exclaimed, "Thank you for looking at me!" Ben immediately turned away,
back to his schedule cards. We had no further contact that day.

Three days later, out of nowhere, Ben looked at me again. Again, I celebrated his noticing me. But this time, he didn't look away. He walked over to me and looked at what I was doing. He said, "You do yours. I do mine." Then he returned to his spot and went back to lining up his cards.

Days later, Ben came over to me, looked at what I was doing, and put his arm around my shoulder. Then he sat down next to me and joined me in lining up my cards. I held my breath and tried not to cry. I couldn't believe it. My baby had come to me. He had chosen to come to me.

By April 2008, almost six months after Ben's diagnosis, I was despondent. The biomedical interventions were producing only superficial improvements in Ben, and no one seemed to have any real answers for us. Then one day, a friend of mine told me she had a cousin in Ireland who had a son Ben's age who had autism. They were running a program there and were seeing meaningful improvements in their son. She encouraged me to look into it. I explained to her I was very busy having a nervous breakdown and that I would look into it later.

It took me six more months of frustration to finally look at the Son-Rise website, but when I finally did, I felt hope again for the first time in months. I immediately had a sense that this new program was different from the other approaches we had tried. Their method seemed compassionate and natural. They said there were no guarantees but that every child had the potential to make amazing progress. I cried while listening to the testimonials of other parents, whose children had recovered. I told my husband I thought this approach might be the answer and that we needed to go for Son-Rise Program training as soon as possible.

Three months later, in December 2008, I attended my first program, the "Start-Up." My mother, a psychotherapist, came with me. At least seventy people attended the program, families of children on the autism spectrum for the most part. Being in the company of other families who shared my situation was profoundly healing. When the teacher made jokes about how "weird" those autistic kids were and how "crazy" some of their behaviors were, we all found ourselves laughing in relief. One teacher talked about a child whose main autistic behavior was reciting entire books of Calvin and Hobbes comic strips. Another talked about a child who hopped, nonstop, for hours. Others talked about kids who smeared poop on the walls, on themselves, and even on their parents. In that room, together, . . . somehow it all seemed funny—even the poop! I laughed one moment, cried the next, and then laughed some more. Things that had felt painful before we came together suddenly didn't feel painful anymore. In that room, we weren't feeling sorry for ourselves or for our children. Everything felt different. We had each other. We had hope.

The Son-Rise Program is a unique, therapeutic, child-centered offering available to families today. The Son-Rise Program is often contrasted with Applied Behavioral Analysis (ABA) and other state-funded therapies, many of which are based on a reward-and-punishment model. The focus in ABA and similar interventions appears to be quantifiable skill acquisition. The Son-Rise Program, on the other hand, focuses on interpersonal-relationship building. The Son-Rise Program inspires a child to want friendships and then teaches him how to establish and sustain them.

The Son-Rise Program also offered us a way for my husband and me, as parents and partners, to heal. This aspect has been terribly important for us, as I don't think we would have had the strength to help Ben if we hadn't been in a simultaneous process of helping ourselves. Ben's challenges were always the main focus, but in order for us to effectively facilitate his Son-Rise Program, my husband and I had to work through the emotional and psychological suffering we had endured during the first five to six years of Ben's life. In other words, we had to address our own special needs before we could successfully address his.

At the end of that first exposure to these new ideas, I decided to place Ben into a full-time Son-Rise Program. This meant we would be working with Ben in our home rather than having him at school with outside therapists. We would now be Ben's teachers and therapists. Accordingly, I came home, and with my mother's support, pulled Ben out of mainstream kindergarten.

Sean, however, was not in agreement with my plan. He was frightened by what he felt, on my part, to be an extreme and impulsive reaction to some very risky new ideas.. He told me I could do as I wished, but warned me, "If it works, it's on you, but if it fails, that's on you, too!" He came around a few months later when we began to see changes in Ben, but his initial reaction was fury toward me and concern for Ben.

I set up a Son-Rise program playroom in our basement and started Ben's program, which we referred to as "homeschool." The playroom is designed to reduce overstimulation, because many children with autism have sensory-processing issues, which means they are often overwhelmed by sounds, etc., that we take for granted. The playroom eliminates overstimulation so that Ben can relax, focus, and interact with other people. It also eliminates control battles—it's a room where he is given control, so we're not having to say no and short circuit the relationship so painstakingly constructed. We started in January 2009 with five to ten hours per week. Four months later, we had worked our way up to nearly forty hours per week.

The first few months were terrible for me. I had no idea what I was doing, and setting up the playroom overwhelmed me. We had to figure out a video camera, shelving, a special, soft linoleum floor—it was all too much. I'm not handy, I can be a perfectionist, and I was terrified that if I didn't do the playroom setup perfectly, Ben wouldn't recover, my husband's doubts would be confirmed, and as usual, it would all be my fault. So I worked like a fiend, sending out flyers for volunteers to come and help us, calling colleges to see if any students wanted to participate in Ben's program, and all the while trying to implement some of the new techniques I had learned. I stressed myself out completely.

But my efforts—as much as I judged them as inadequate—were, in the end, sufficient. Within months of implementing our program, we began to see exciting changes in Ben. For the first time in his life, he began to actually choose to connect with us. Language, which had always been garbled and never a means of communication, now became a tool for Ben to interact with us. He showed more eye contact. We were cautiously hopeful.

For the next three years, I oversaw Ben's full-time Son-Rise Program in our home. To build our team of facilitators who would be working in shifts, one-on-one with Ben, on a daily basis, I initially found volunteers, then paid hired workers, and ultimately hired au pairs, who were in this country for the sole purpose of caring for my children. Our au pairs had no previous special-needs experience, but they were enthusiastic and open to learning and that was enough for me. Additionally, as we ran Ben's Son-Rise Program, I continued to explore a variety of biomedical interventions to heal Ben's body as well as his mind. Today, I understand how intricately connected his body and his behavior truly are.

Three years later, Ben was unrecognizable. The boy who had no idea we were in the room with him was fully invested in relationships and deeply desirous of friends and connections. Moreover, Ben wasn't the only one who had changed. Through running our Son-Rise Program and developing our own interpersonal skills, the entire family transformed into much more loving, self-aware, expressive, and happy people.

OUR EARLY SON-RISE PROGRAM YEARS

In many ways, our initial Son-Rise Program period, from January 2009 until the fall of 2011, was the most rigorous and transformational period of our entire journey, because it was during this period that Ben truly emerged from his isolation and allowed us to connect with him—for the first time in his life. These first three years were tough, powerful, and, at times, painful. We were in a crucible, and Ben's development was our golden reward.

We began our full-time Son-Rise Program in April 2009, with multiple hours each day, including weekends, of Son-Rise Program playroom time. Initially, we got volunteers from colleges and special-education graduate programs to work with Ben, but for the most part, they were unreliable (this one graduated, that one moved, that one got pregnant, that one fell off the face of the earth, etc.), so we began to hire people, from resources like SitterCity, Craigslist, and anywhere else I could find them.

Eventually we hired au pairs, who lived with us, had a consistent schedule, and were focused entirely on helping Ben and supporting the rest of the family. Setting up the playroom, hiring au pairs, and leaving behind income-generating work so that I could devote my time 100 percent to Ben's program, as well as to the care of my daughter, caused financial strain for us. But we decided at the outset that we would rather pay for Ben's recovery now, and possibly *heal* him, than pay to *manage* Ben's autism for the rest of our lives.

We ran our full-time Son-Rise Program for almost three years. Some weeks we spent as much as forty to fifty hours in the playroom, and other weeks much less, more like fifteen to twenty. We realized that although spending time in the playroom was central to Ben's growth, the crucial issue was not, for us, the number of hours spent in the playroom, but rather the quality and maintenance of our "Son-Rise Program Attitude" ("the Attitude"), which we learned during our program courses. Essentially, the Attitude means being nonjudgmental, totally present, and totally loving and wanting the best for Ben. We learned to see ourselves, in all of our interactions with Ben, as "ambassadors for the human race." We learned to be "user-friendly," and to constantly employ the Three E's: energy, excitement, and enthusiasm. I learned not to need a particular behavior or progress from Ben in order to be happy. Having such a need inadvertently puts pressure on our kids, which they resist strongly. We learned to "choose happiness" for ourselves, because we were role models for Ben, and we wanted him to choose happiness in his own life. Ironically, over the years, Ben's consistent ability to choose happiness, even in the face of grave disappointments and heartfelt emotional wounds, taught *me* more than I ever taught him about choosing happiness!

We practiced the Attitude on a daily basis in our home, to the best of our ability. My husband and I practiced it with both children, as well as with each other. We realized, at a certain point, that our entire home had in fact become one great big Son-Rise Program playroom! We were all free to play, to express our authentic feelings, and to be ourselves—without judgment. As a family, through our Son-Rise Program experience during those first few years, we transformed as much as Ben did.

When we started our program, Ben was initially resistant to his Son-Rise Program playroom. But within weeks, Ben developed a desire, an enjoyment, and ultimately a need for his playroom time. In the playroom, the child is completely in control. Apart from any obviously destructive behavior, he is allowed to do what he likes and is never wrong. If Ben said the sky was green with yellow polka dots, it was. If Ben wanted to tear paper for hours and hours, we tore paper until he was done. If Ben wanted to play *his* game, we played it. If Ben wanted to have nothing to do with us, we let go and stayed present but gave him space to do his own thing.

We went *with* Ben, and with his "isms" (exclusive and repetitive behaviors), instead of trying to make him do what we wanted him to do. Rewards and punishments were not part of the playroom. Over time, *Ben's relationship with us* became the reward, as our presence in the playroom was full of the Three E's. We showed Ben, through our nonjudgmental and consistently loving and fun attitudes, that other people were "user-friendly" and safe.

We worked on social goals rather than academic ones. These goals were eye contact, flexibility, communication, and interactive–attention span (the measure of how long Ben could engage in activities with others without a break). We kept in mind that we were modeling for him the social skills he would need when he eventually went to school.

We also learned through our Son-Rise Program that media (*e.g.*, television, computers, any iThings) exacerbated Ben's autism, so we eliminated them 100 percent from Ben's life.

On a daily basis, we brought in games we created with built-in social goals. If Ben was doing autism, and choosing not to interact with us, we would then "join" him. In other words, we gave him space, both physically and figuratively, to do the activity he wanted to do. We ourselves did the *same* activity he did, not with an intention to get him to want to be with us, but rather to understand him better through engaging in the activity he was clearly finding so interesting and fun (*i.e.*, his ism). If Ben drew mazes for hours, we drew mazes for hours. If Ben wandered around the room, feeling the texture of the wall as he went, we did the same. Joining is kind of like when you and a friend are hanging out together, both maybe reading or on your laptops, not interacting directly or maybe only occasionally, but the experience is more fun because you are together, even though you're not doing the activity together.

As we joined Ben, if for even a fleeting moment Ben looked at us, or even toward us, we "celebrated" the look with great cheers, delight, and enthusiasm, by verbalizing our excitement at his choice to connect or even jumping up and down enthusiastically.

If, on the other hand, Ben chose to be interactive during a session, we engaged with him in whatever way he wanted. He chose the game we played, not us. If he wanted to play *his* game, we played that. The purpose was not to "teach" him, but to *connect* with him, with no agenda other than to love him and demonstrate to him that he could handle the interaction.

I struggled terribly with our Son-Rise Program for much of the first three years. Hours in the playroom often flew by for many of Ben's Son-Rise Program Child Facilitators, but not for me. I had an inferiority complex about my mothering abilities, and I constantly forgot to hold a nonjudgmental attitude toward myself. I was my own worst enemy in the playroom. I worried that I was boring, unloving, and selfish. I didn't *want* to sit around for an hour or so and join Ben in his autism, and I was ashamed of my resistance.

Over phone and Skype consultations, I talked about my feelings with a teacher at the Autism Treatment Center of America*, where the Son-Rise Program is taught. He helped me identify my feelings, and in so doing, realize where I was holding on to certain beliefs that engendered those feelings. He helped me to recognize that my resistance was because I was terrified. I believed that I, alone, was responsible for Ben's recovery, and that if Ben remained autistic, both my life and my family's lives would be terrible. I feared his autism, and being face to face with it in the playroom meant being face-to-face with my fears. So the playroom was unbearable for me. Outwardly, I was supposed

---

* Since 1983, the Autism Treatment Center of America, sited at the Option Institute, has provided innovative training programs for parents and professionals caring for children challenged by Autism, Autism Spectrum Disorders, Pervasive Developmental Disorder (PDD), and other developmental difficulties. Over 25,000 families have been helped by *The Son-Rise Program*. For more information, visit www.autismtreatmentcenter.org.

to be practicing the Attitude, loving unconditionally, not judging, and all the rest, but inside I felt bored, guilty, and ashamed of my feelings. I was supposed to be the mentor for everyone on our Son-Rise Program team! In my mind, I was a total fake.

Working with my Son-Rise Program teacher, however, I was ultimately able to let go of many of my fears and negative beliefs. But it took me years. I eventually realized that I was not responsible for Ben's recovery, any more than I was responsible for the outcome of the life of any other person in my family. I wanted to go for the brass ring, so I was going to give it my all for Ben's recovery. But if he didn't recover, I could still love him, and we could still have a decent life. I just had to let go of my agenda for that life and start practicing happiness with where we were at that moment—including Ben's still-autistic condition.

My experience in the playroom radically improved over time, but I can't emphasize enough how hard it was for me to learn to love and accept Ben as he was and myself as I was. The Son-Rise Program taught me how to love. But in some ways, seeing my own inability to love—both Ben as well as myself—was a revelation that showed me where my work truly lay. Today I'm grateful, but back then it was very tough.

During this period, we envisioned Ben well, recovered, having friends, being in school, participating in activities, and connecting with the world and its inhabitants. By far, the most meaningful gain we saw by the end of the first few years was Ben's revolutionary desire to connect with others. On a biomedical level, however, we still had not found the right "recipe," and continued to see autistic symptoms on a regular basis. But eventually, the work of the first few years planted a seed of connection in Ben, which later blossomed within him to enable him to establish meaningful, substantive, and fulfilling relationships with others.

BLOGGING OUR EARLY SON-RISE YEARS

My blog started out as a vehicle to document our family history and share our process with family and friends. Over time, however, the blog became an integral tool in my self-care kit. As I wrote each night, I expressed and assessed my feelings from the day, analyzed Ben's status, and documented changes in our biomedical protocols. As people began to follow my writing online and offer comments, I felt less and less alone, especially in the realization that many of the readers were from foreign countries, where autism had also imposed itself on their families.

Some of the blog postings are, I have been told, inspirational and moving. Others are comical. Some are sad, and others are heartbreaking. Some postings are emotionally raw, humbling, and embarrassing to me. I include this last category because I wish to illustrate my fallibility and convey the message that parental perfection is not required for a child to make meaningful progress. You feel what you feel, but you keep going, you keep trying to help your child. Every posting is an authentic snapshot of a moment in our life at some point during the past six years. The entire collection is an album of moments, moments that ultimately culminated in Ben's immense progress and his liberation from a world of acute isolation.

One thing I wish to note about the postings is that throughout the process, I tried to absorb the principles I was learning. As I read over some of the postings now, I hear myself trying to persuade myself that the principles, some of which I initially found very hard to accept, actually make sense or at least resonate within me on some level. So as you read the postings, please understand that I am trying to believe in the new ideas I am learning, in the hope that believing in these principles will help Ben. Thus if my words come off saccharine at times—or perhaps a little too much—you will now, I hope, understand why.

SATURDAY, DECEMBER 19, 2009

We have always known that our children are miracles. But because of our new attitude, we no longer wait for Ben to be cured to enjoy him and live our lives. Life is not a dress rehearsal. Parenting isn't about waiting for Ben to be recovered. We trust and hope that Ben will be off the spectrum completely one day. We don't know when it will happen, just that it can happen. But we are learning to love without judgment right now—both of our children and each other—and it is changing us.

Changes in Ben so far:

Over the past nine to ten months that we have been running our Son-Rise Program, Ben has moved from an isolated, disconnected, and remote child into a child who is starting to connect regularly with us. We spend six to ten hours every day in his Son-Rise Program play-room, a distraction-free environment we built in the basement, where we play with Ben one-on-one. We enjoy him, and he enjoys us.

WEDNESDAY, DECEMBER 30, 2009

Our Son-Rise Program team and I spend hours every day with Ben in his Son-Rise Program playroom. With very few toys or other objects to distract Ben, and always only one person at a time in the room with him, the focus of our play is Ben's relationship with the person with him in the room at that time.

Autism is a social disorder, so our curriculum with Ben is social, rather than academic. Regular kids need to learn reading, 'riting, and 'rithmetic. But Ben needs to learn how to interact socially, and that's what we work on. The four fundamentals in his social curriculum are eye contact, communication, flexibility, and interactive–attention span. We use games to target goals within each of these fundamental areas.

Once a month we assess Ben's progress. We examine what skills we need to work on. We use it to generate goals for our team to focus on, and this month we have three specific goals:

1. We will encourage Ben to speak slowly and clearly.
2. We will inspire Ben to allow central variations to his games (central variations are changes to his game that substantially alter the direction of the game).
3. We will inspire Ben to hold sustained eye contact for seven-second increments.

SUNDAY, JANUARY 3, 2010

An *ism*, in Son-Rise Program vernacular, refers to an activity that is both exclusive and repetitive, such as spinning plates, circuiting a room repeatedly, or most frequent for Ben, telling the same story repeatedly without any interaction with others. In the past, Ben's ism-ing was terrifying to me, because I judged it, I judged him, and I judged myself. I am starting to realize, however, that I don't have to be afraid of Ben's autism. If Ben's autism is part of him, and I hate and fear his autism, then I hate and fear a fundamental part of him. Today I am trying to embrace his autism, with its attendant isms, as a way for Ben to take care of himself. Ism-ing allows Ben time to process the world. His brain needs that time. I'm starting to get that now.

Ben's main ism is storytelling. He tells the same stories, with the same characters, over and over, for hours on end. There are variations on the plots, and sometimes he changes the characters, but it's basically the same stuff, over and over, for literally hours and hours. Ben and I told stories last night from 5:30 PM until he fell asleep at 9:30 PM. This morning we told stories from when he woke up at 6:30 AM until 11:00 AM, when my first session ended.

We told stories again this afternoon from 1:45 to 3:00, during our second session.

Less than a year ago, after a weekend like this one, I'd probably be wrecked by now. Instead, I consider that I spent this weekend deeply connecting with Ben. I speak his language—storytelling—because that's the way he is able to connect. So he wasn't telling me about his favorite Red Sox player, and he wasn't tell me about his school science fair. But he was *with me*, and I was *with him*. It just has to be on his terms. Life is not a dress rehearsal, and I will never get these moments back. I want to use them to love and connect with my son. So I will continue to speak Ben's language as long as that is the language he chooses.

Many moments these days, almost a year into our Son-Rise Program, he chooses to speak our language. But in the moments when he doesn't, I'm grateful that I don't need him to be anyone other than who he is.

Oops, here he comes. "Mommy, can I tell you a story?" "Ben, I'd love to hear it!"

The Specific Carbohydrate Diet

Ben is on the Specific Carbohydrate Diet (SCD), which eliminates all yeast-feeding food residue from his gut. Yeast is one of the biggest villains in our autism comic book, and going on SCD has led to great progress for Ben in the areas of ism-ing and eye contact. The problem with the diet is that it is basically a part-time job—every food must be cooked from scratch—and as I repeatedly comment to friends, "I can't even buy Whole Foods unsweetened applesauce!" Also, Ben is a picky eater, so many textures and new foods are repugnant to him. (Alina is also on SCD, because of a stomach problem she has experienced since she was an infant.)

When we started SCD in July 2009, I dived in. I submerged myself in the new recipes and cooking, grinding almonds, food processing vegetables, frying pancakes made with bananas and eggs, steaming chicken, turkey, beef, and pork, slow-cooking apples for applesauce, searching for "SCD-legal" juices, juicing fruits, baking muffins, baking brownies, baking cupcakes—all concocted with ingredients like nuts, meats, vegetables, and eggs, ingredients hidden inside apparently palatable and somewhat everyday-looking foods. Things like muffins made with chicken, and pudding made with avocados. For weeks I cooked for six to eight hours a day.

I experimented endlessly and finally discovered a few foods that Ben was willing to eat. We told the children they had "buggies" in their tummies (*i.e.*, yeast), and that they could only eat foods that "the buggies didn't like." So the nut cookies were renamed "bug-hate bagels." The nut-and-winter-squash brownies were renamed "bug-hate brownies." Every time the children want a food, they ask, "Mommy, do the buggies like this food?" Most times, unfortunately, the answer is yes for the buggies, and no for the kids.

After months of this cooking tidal wave, I began to train our babysitter to prepare a lot of the foods. She took on much of the cooking, under my supervision. I felt reborn. She went on vacation one weekend, and I found myself back in the kitchen, for almost four hours, baking brownies, cookies, and honey bread (made with chicken, eggs, honey, and other non-yeast-causing ingredients). It was exhausting, and I was exceedingly grateful when she returned.

Croissants and autism

Ben is currently in a "mode," and has been that way for weeks. A "mode" refers to a return to autistic symptoms due to a changing brain. The Son-Rise Program taught us to see a mode not as a sign of regression, but rather as a "time out" for a brain that has made some progress and needs some time to assimilate the changes.

I remember another time when Ben suddenly returned to this kind of lack of interest and spaced-out stuff—it was before we went on SCD. Ben had been on a gluten-free/casein-free diet for seven months when I attempted to reintroduce gluten, in the form of a croissant, one of his favorite foods, to reward him for something. For the next three to four days, Ben demonstrated autistic symptoms the likes of which we hadn't seen for six to seven months. He was like a zombie. Then, suddenly, after three or four days, he snapped back to the much more interactive and present kid we had gotten used to. Apparently the gluten was out of his system. The experience convinced us that gluten is a problem, and we've never gone back.

MONDAY, JANUARY 11, 2010

Today, after a reasonable night's sleep and a bit more perspective, I think Ben's mode, which has happily ended, may have been symptoms of a negative "biomedical" reaction to too many apples. Apples are one of a number of foods that contain high amounts of phenols, chemicals that give color to foods and other things in the environment, and that cause problems for many autistic children. We have been giving Ben much more of these foods for the past few weeks, ever since I bought a fancy popsicle machine that uses apple juice—oops! So we are removing these high-phenol food items from Ben's diet, effective immediately. In addition, we heard back from our SCD nutritionist, and are going to prepare nut yogurt and a bunch of new SCD recipes.

Two days later

Amazingly, Sean thinks Ben is "waking up" out of the ism-ing already—after only one day without the high-phenol foods. It really seems that overdosing on apples, green grapes, and fruit juice engendered this re-surgence of ism-ing in Ben. How wonderful to be paying attention so we can make helpful adjustments! Also, Sean had the great idea of using other, nonphenolic fruits for Ben to make popsicles and other treats.

THURSDAY, JANUARY 28, 2010

Weeks later

Wow, wow, wow. Who knows if it was a mode, bad reaction to the fruit, or what, but Ben has clearly emerged from it and has apparently taken a quantum leap in the past week! There is no doubt that re-moving the high-phenol fruits (apples and grapes) from his diet vastly diminished his need for constant ism-ing. Ben is currently responsive, interested, funny, and flexible. His eye contact is completely sponta-neous and nearly neurotypical, including sustained eye contact for five to six seconds at a time, which has been one of our goals. We had a last-minute schedule change yesterday and had to flip the times of two homeschool teachers. Ben was comfortable and flexible with the changed schedule, despite the schedule sign hung that morning in the playroom with a different lineup. A penny has definitely dropped.

Die-off

Ben's withdrawal from the high-phenol foods is proving challenging, however. Tonight he cried all evening, and he has been manic and moody for the past two days. We have seen this before, when he went off other foods he couldn't tolerate. But I felt happy anyway. I didn't even feel like I was *choosing* to be happy. I just felt happy to be with him—as we sang thirty-five to forty children's songs on the acron-ymed list he created during the day and felt the need to go through between 9:30 and 10:00 PM. I am also noticing that *my choice to be happy seems to have a calming effect on Ben.*

Ben has entered a new stage. His eye contact at times seems almost neurotypical—spontaneous, consistent, and sustained, which is incredible to me. His interactive communication has also improved—he doesn't miss a beat. He yelled out something from another room this afternoon, to correct something someone had said. Then tonight he wanted to sell something in the house to raise money to purchase a toy he wants. Sean exclaimed, "Well, we can't sell Alina!" and Ben responded with, "No, because I love her very, very much!"

Ben is a miracle, unfolding before my eyes.

THURSDAY, MARCH 4, 2010

Horrible the Horse!

Today Ben told me a short story he made up about a horse named Horrible. Horrible did everything wrong, intentionally, and had three horse friends, who did everything right. Ben focused more on the three good friends than on Horrible. I'm so proud of him. The story title is fantastic, and Ben's take on *The Tale of Peter Rabbit*, one of our favorite stories, is a great innovation. One of Ben's favorite games is taking a book he has read only moments ago and rewriting it with new characters, typically characters from his playroom or from other favorite books he has previously read. It seems to be a way of taking someone else's story into his personal world, but with inhabitants *he* chooses. Perhaps it gives him a sense of control.

I am deepening my commitment to our Son-Rise Program journey. I quit my part-time job, which I have had for more than seven years and enjoyed immensely. I am spending more time on the development of Son-Rise Program games, more time in the playroom, and more time with my daughter. I am moving closer to where I want to be, which is with my children and not running away from them as I used to. We are blessed that Sean earns enough to support us and that our family is also helping out. It's hard to take hand outs, but Ben needs us to be willing to do so.

When we got the autism diagnosis, I told Sean that God was calling me back to our children. This is more true today than ever before in my time as a mother. I want to be with them now. Perhaps I always did but was too afraid I would fail at the task. God knew better.

SATURDAY, MARCH 20, 2010

I came home from a week-long Son-Rise Program course last night. In the past, when I have gone away for any length of time, Ben showed little emotion upon my return, and I got used to expecting no reaction. He gave me, at best, a brief hello, at worst, total disinterest.

Last night, however, Ben gave me a gift I will never forget. I was tucking him in. I kissed him and was about to say good night and leave the room, when Ben suddenly said, "Mommy, I'm glad you're home." My heart leaped. "Really, Ben?" I exclaimed. Then he said, "I missed you."

I can't tell you the joy I felt in that moment. My son, the love of my heart, expressing honest and authentic love for me, unexpected and unsolicited. "I missed you too, Ben," I whispered.

SATURDAY, MARCH 27, 2010

My little manipulator!

This afternoon Ben and Alina were fighting over which chapter to read in an Oliver the Pig book. Ben wanted chapter three, Alina chapter one. I told them, "Guess what number is in my head. Whoever guesses closest gets to choose the chapter!" Ben guessed forty. Alina guessed three. The number was one. Ben became upset and frustrated and said, "No, I get to choose!" I responded, "No, Ben, that's not fair. Alina won, and she gets to choose." Alina said, "Yes, and I want chapter one!"

Ben leaped off my lap, ran to the sofa, buried his head in his hands, and moaned, with one eye peeking out, "Mommy, I don't want to play with you anymore!" I said, "Well, Ben, I'm sad, but Alina still gets to choose." Happily for me, Alina had by that time realized it was dinner time and yelled out, "It's okay, Mommy, Ben can choose, it's dinner time." Ben ran back to my lap, and we read chapter three.

So here's the miracle (among the thousands I won't go into, having to do with Ben conversing with us, Ben negotiating, Ben noticing us, Ben looking at us): *Ben tried to manipulate me.* Like any normal, healthy, neurotypical seven-year-old would. Rather than getting stuck in a self-centered, rigid rant, demanding his way in the situation with no awareness of anything other than getting what he wanted, Ben actually was aware of me and my feelings, and tried to manipulate the situation by manipulating *my feelings*. He was *aware of me* and tried to create an emotion in me in order to get me to give him what he wanted. "Mommy, I don't want to play with you anymore!"

I am happy, happy, *happy.* The most wonderful part: I'm happy because I'm loving my child—not because of his progress. I'm happy because I'm not missing out—not because of his progress. I'm happy because I have decided to be happy—*and I love his progress.*

MONDAY, APRIL 5, 2010

Loving Ben's Autism

This morning I had a realization. About fourteen years ago, I had a car accident. It left me with seemingly incurable upper-back pain for almost six years. The pain was acute and constant. It wreaked havoc on my relationships, my self-esteem, and my job.

Two years after the accident, I became engaged to be married. My fiancé (now my husband) and I entered into premarital counseling with the rabbi who was to marry us. One week, the rabbi gave us a questionnaire about our relationship. We had to fill them out separately, and we were not allowed to see each other's answers before our next meeting with the rabbi. At our next session, we reviewed the questionnaire. One of the questions was, "What do you hate most about your partner?" The rabbi asked Sean what he had written. Sean replied instantly: "Susan's back."

I sucked in hard, feeling kicked in the guts. I felt angry, hurt, and humiliated, and tears filled my eyes. Although I was aware that my back pain caused tremendous problems in our relationship, hearing Sean say he actually hated my back devastated me. It took me many years, even after my back healed, to let go of the sadness I felt upon learning that Sean felt that way. Because my back was a part of *me*, challenged or not.

This morning I was mulling over the idea that loving Ben means loving his autism. I wondered out loud, "Do I really believe that?" I wanted to be honest with myself. Suddenly I remembered my feelings when Sean told me he hated my back. I remembered the hurt I felt, because he hated a part of me. Ben would feel just as hurt, I suddenly realized, if he knew—and I believe he has known, on some level—that I hated and feared his autism. Because, like my back, his autism is part of *him*, limiting and challenging or not. Today I want to love Ben, love his autism, and love all of my child—because it's all part of him, and *I want to love him*. It's my choice. I get to decide.

Love is the absence of judgment. Love is the acceptance and embrace of the whole person, as he or she shows up now, in this moment. I get it now. It's liberation from fear, control, worry, and judgment—a true experience of love.

I have such an eraser brain that I actually often forget what it used to be like before Ben started to come out of his autistic world. I forget that he almost never looked at us, never talked to us, usually didn't seem to hear us, most of the time didn't seem to care if we were there or not. Now his grumpy faces if I'm taking too long to get off the phone to read him a story, his joyful game playing with us, his unsolicited hugs and kisses, and his total-dead-on eye contact when I kiss him goodnight—these are all commonplace. But I forget that it has only been a few *months* that Ben has been so connected and expressive. Just months.

TUESDAY, MAY 4, 2010

Ben yelled tonight. Ben has never yelled. *Ever.* He has thrown tantrums, whined, and cried, all very loudly at times. But when we have asked him to yell at the top of his lungs (for some good purpose), he hasn't done it. When we ask Ben to "shout it out, honey, give it to me loud!" his "shout" comes out just barely audible.

But tonight—ho, ho! Ben was upstairs, and Sean asked him to say goodnight to our au pair, Oscar. Ben said in his usual way, that is, slightly louder than under his breath, "Good night, Oscar." But when Sean then asked, "Ben, say goodnight, but louder," Ben *shouted,* "Good night, Oscar!" Sean ran into the bedroom, where I sat working, his face lit up with joy. "Did you hear that?" I answered, my face lit up with the same happy amazement, "Absolutely, yes! *Oh my God*, Sean!"

SATURDAY, MAY 22, 2010

The Son-Rise Program was founded by Samahria Kaufman and her husand Barry Neil Kaufman. During one of our Son-Rise Program courses,

Samahria said to me, "A happy woman is a woman who completely loves herself exactly the way she is. That's the only real Son-Rise mom!" Feeling good about myself doesn't come naturally to me. I easily focus on what I should do better and the ways in which I fall short. Others see such good in me, and yet I struggle with core feelings of inadequacy. But I'm trying to be a good mother and that counts for something—even to me.

I dearly pray for Ben to be fully off the spectrum at some point in the next few years, and to graduate from his Son-Rise Program. But life is always a choice to be happy or unhappy, to be grateful or self-pitying, to be present or run away. So I know when Ben is off the spectrum, we will have new challenges. We're building strong happiness-choosing muscles in our life each day, right now, so whatever life brings now and later, we can make the choice to be happy each moment with the help of God. I am not a victim of circumstances; I am the active captain of my attitude—and for today I choose an attitude of gratitude.

Autistic symptoms back again

Observations of Ben from the past few days:

1. He has been laughing nonsensically frequently throughout the day, particularly in the morning and at mealtimes. He used to do this a lot; it's a typical autistic behavior. It had diminished to almost never, but now we are seeing a lot of it. It's associated, like so many symptoms that we call autism, with yeast overgrowth.

2. He has been more rigid and inflexible the past few days as well. He would not share his new game with Alina this evening, he would not compromise about what videos to watch last night, and he would not help with cleanup this evening or earlier today. He is usually very willing to help clean up.

3. He has been more demanding, by far, and slightly more aggressive than normal (*i.e.*, the last few months).

The timing of these behaviors coincides with the start of a supplement we are trying called oxytocin, so we need to keep an eye on it. But he has also been doing too many activities, in my opinion, and this is somewhat owing to my eagerness to give him some "typical summer fun." But Ben's not *typical.*

I have to be more patient.

SUNDAY, MAY 30, 2010

Ben has taken another leap forward. In Sean's words, "He's making concise, intelligent statements without hesitation or pause in order to process. We're having intelligent conversations, about other people, in fact, such as Alina. This afternoon we discussed possibilities for consequences when Alina lies, and we asked Ben for input. He suggested various things; some made sense and some didn't. When we decided on four days without peas (her favorite vegetable) and we asked Ben if it was a good idea, he grinned and said, 'Yes!' And it's happening consistently, today and yesterday."

We are grateful for the progress, but I am happy mostly because I get to be with Ben and he is revealing more of himself to us all the time. We are learning on the Alina front as well, to be more clear and comfortable and to enforce consequences with her, which is hard for me. I worry that she sees a double standard in how we treat Ben versus how we treat her. We hold her accountable for things we don't require of Ben, because she is able to function at a higher level in so many areas. It's not fair, and we all know it.

WEDNESDAY, JUNE 30, 2010

Old scene, old Ben; old scene, new Ben!

In the past, Ben refused to go onto a playground if even one other child was there before him or if another kid entered after he did. He would shake, walk backward, cry, and totally freak out until we left. "I need to go home; I need to go home," he would rail. The behavior started after Ben attended a camp for children with special needs two summers ago, before we knew Ben had autism. We still don't know what happened, but one day Ben just stopped being willing to go on playgrounds if other kids were there. It was very painful.

This evening, Sean took Ben to a park near a playground to try out a new four-wheeled scooter Sean had bought for Ben. Ben did pretty well and worked really hard despite some challenges with balancing. Afterward, Sean tried to take Ben onto the playground, and Ben resisted in his usual fashion. But Sean observed some key differences.

First of all, Ben was willing to try something new and different (the scooter) and was even excited about it! Then, at the park, while Sean was showing him the scooter and how to ride it, Ben listened to Sean and tried to follow instructions on how to position his feet so that he could actually ride the scooter. Next, when Sean tried to take Ben to the playground, although Ben refused to go on because there were two other children already there (two five-year-olds), Ben didn't shut down the way he used to, that is, with panic and crying. Instead, he was willing to *explain* to Sean that the presence of the two children was causing him discomfort and that if they left he would be willing to go on the playground.

Further, when Sean offered Ben a possible solution (*i.e.,* asking the children to leave the playground), Ben declined his offer "because that would make the children cry." In other words, Ben was concerned for the children's emotional states. *And*, Ben was responsive to Sean's question.

Next, Sean offered another solution, which was that Sean ask the children's brother, who was playing nearby, to ask the children to move. Showing real flexibility, Ben responded, "Yes, that would be okay." Sean actually ended up explaining the situation to the parents, who were also nearby, and they got their children to go just outside of the playground. Once the children had left, Ben was willing to go on the playground.

In addition, Ben also made two comments during his discussion with Sean:

1. If Alina had been there, she could have asked the children to leave, and
2. Ben was afraid to go on the playground, because he didn't know the children's names.

Ben has never explained #2 to us before. He also said that if he did know their names, he would be willing to go on. *So Ben's refusal to go on the playground with other children was based on the fact that they were strangers.* How amazing that Ben shared that piece of his process!

After going briefly on the playground, Sean and Ben went back to the scooter. Ben watched Sean ride the scooter and then tried riding himself. Sean held the handlebars so that Ben wouldn't have to worry about his balance but could just practice keeping both feet on the scooter, and they rode back to the car that way. Ben focused on the shadows more than anything else, and he never stopped talking to Sean.

Old scene, old Ben. Old Ben didn't talk. Old Ben shut down and didn't have words or apparent desire to express his internal process. Old Ben did not respond to solutions offered to him. Old Ben did not respond, period.

Old scene, new Ben. New Ben talked. New Ben did not shut down despite fear. New Ben communicated with Daddy about his desires and his feelings, and accepted solutions.

Ben tells us more of who he is now, and what his experience is, moment by moment. It's easy for some children, but not for ours. Our child is climbing a mountain. We're all climbing it together: Ben, Sean and I, and Alina, too. We hit some beautiful views along the way.

TUESDAY, JULY 6, 2010

Ben had a full-on tantrum today, because he wanted me to get a CD player so we could practice a dance. Electronics of any kind are not allowed in the playroom. Because I have learned to see aggression in Ben as a form of communication, I was able to stay light and easy when he went into the tantrum and to actually have fun. Ben pulled out all the stops, doing everything he could to get me to change my mind, including knocking over chairs, throwing things, biting me, crying, and whining. He even announced, "I'm going to do naughty things!"

Ben told me that he wanted to go upstairs, so we could dance, and that he wanted homeschool to be over so we could go upstairs. I stayed happy, light, and comfortable, and he was visibly frustrated by my lack of engagement in a power struggle. He yelled, "You *are* upset, Mommy!" I replied, "No, I'm really happy just to be with you, and you can cry or do whatever you need to do, and I will just stay with you and love you!"

47

Then he pointed to the chairs he had just knocked over, "It's not okay with you, Mommy!" I laughed and said, "Actually, everything's okay with me, honey!" Then he tried to bite me. I gently drew my hand away and asked him if he wanted something else to bite. After a few more unsuccessful attempts to provoke me, Ben yelled, "If you don't let me go upstairs, I will be always hurting someone!" I smiled and replied, "I understand." Finally, Ben ended up trying to scare me and saying "Boo! Boo!" I answered in a silly, exaggerated way, "Eek! No! Don't scare me! Eek!"

Eventually he pooped out and sat on the floor. At that point, I put on some silly glasses and pretended to be a goofy person looking for a boy named Benjamin, and made a joke about the air conditioner being a monster. Ben ended up laughing hysterically about the air conditioner "monster" and wet his pants. So I went and got new pants and some juice for Ben. That was the end of the tantrum.

Afterwards, Ben went into a rigid game* he created. I didn't offer any challenges. Notably, when the next homeschool teacher entered with a funny game, Ben was happy and responsive. He had moved on and totally let go of what had gone before.

SATURDAY, AUGUST 7, 2010

Progress sound bites 1

- Today Ben imitated my language. He said, "Hell-o-o!!" in response to my saying something jokingly wrong.
- Sean presented Dinosaur Bingo to Ben today. Ben wanted to play. He and Ben and Alina took turns spinning the spinner, and Ben played right along, the whole way through.

---

* A rigid game in the Son-Rise Program refers to a game in which the child interacts with a facilitator but demands complete control of the entire interaction, with no allowance for flexibility of any kind.

- This evening, when Sean came down to see what was going on with the kids (we were up in the loft for our movie night while the kids were downstairs for their TV night), Ben came over, looked Sean right in the eye, and said, "Daddy, can we have one more show? Pleeeeeeease?"

- This afternoon, Ben suddenly ran out into the yard. I quickly ran after him, thinking he was going to turn on the hose. When I called out, "Ben, I can't see you!" he responded with, "I'm over here, bringing in my toys to the house!" And he was. He had left toys outside while playing earlier and had come outside to clean them up!

- When Sean came down earlier today, Ben had invented "Chocolate Checkers," and asked, "Who will play with me?" Later, he wanted to play with Alina and invented a new game for her.

- He had terrific eye contact, unsolicited and continuous.

- Ben took a huge nap this afternoon, which has resulted in it being 9:15 PM and him still awake. So I went in to say a second goodnight, and Ben looked at me, grinned, and said, "Mommy? God woke me up and told me a Mickey Mouse story." Full eye contact, huge grin.

- He spent time today with me doing a workbook sheet, unscrambling letters on road signs. He is becoming extremely cooperative in doing academic work, such as reading and workbook exercises.

- We spent the afternoon with Sean's parents today, in part to celebrate the upcoming birthday of Sean's mother, Grandma Ro. Ben participated fully in helping write a card to Grandma Ro (though the letter was actually on the envelope), and when it came time to present our gift and sing happy birthday, Ben was completely present and happy to participate.

For the first time, I am finding myself able to envision Ben eventually in an academic-school setting. We are a long way from that point, certainly, but it is looking possible for the first time. Thy will be done.

WEDNESDAY, AUGUST 11, 2010

Progress sound bites 2

- I made coconut-egg pancakes for the childrens' breakfast today. When I asked Ben if he liked them, he looked directly at me and responded, "Yes, Mommy, because you made them. That's why I like them."
- He is picking things up and putting messes on tables rather than just throwing it unconsciously onto the floor.
- He is eating more foods than ever before.
- He asked me to find new people for his Son-Rise Program— he wants more contact with others.
- He is more expressive of his love for others than ever before.

He is exactly where he is supposed to be, and I am just grateful that he is Ben—in whatever way he chooses to be with us.

THURSDAY, AUGUST 12, 2010

Ben wowed me again today.

He was not only willing to go through another, entire, grade-1 activity book, but additionally, as one of the exercises in the book, he was willing to do a color-by-numbers page of three fish. Ben has never, *ever*, ever been willing, interested, or, possibly, able to color by numbers.

At the end of our session, when the next person entered the room to play with Ben, Ben said to her, "Come back later!" She replied, "Well, Ben, it's my turn now." I added, "Yes, Ben, I have to go run an errand now." Ben then replied, "Oh, okay, then you can help me instead!" I wildly celebrated his flexibility and thanked him for playing with me. I ran up here to the kitchen, filled with excitement.

His handwriting is a disaster.

He insists on changing words into his own language.

He is obsessed with words and objects of his own creation, that have no bearing on reality.

He is still out of context much of the time.

WHO CARES!!!

THURSDAY, AUGUST 19, 2010

This week, Ben went for his glutathione* shot. The appointment involved three events, as follows.

Ben's communication style is much more that of a normal child these days. Something about his tone, and that his words are not so drawn out and formal. He also is not laughing without any reason anymore, which is a shift from just two weeks ago!

Today in the playroom, I tried to teach Ben how to tell time. Rather than using a theme, however, I tried to use the First Grade Activities Book we're going through, and Ben shut down. I tried to get him to do it for about ten minutes, at the end of which Ben ended up just staring into space. I realized I had focused too much on an academic goal rather than a social goal, and I felt uncomfortable.

---

* Glutathione is a tripeptide in our brain, which is used by practically every cell in the body to neutralize toxins. Children with autism typically have insufficient levels of glutathione, and many of the biomedical interventions serve to increase glutathione levels (*e.g.*, hyperbaric oxygen therapy, dietary interventions, etc.). Ben gets an IV shot of glutathione every four to six weeks. The shots have resulted in visibly stronger eye contact and mental clarity.

I judged myself because I hadn't created any new themes lately, and because my focus, now that Ben is less autistic, had shifted onto academics and away from having a Son-Rise Program Attitude. It was a good learning experience.

On a wonderful note, Ben's eye contact today, especially when we went upstairs for him to use the bathroom, was great. His huge blue eyes amaze me.

MONDAY, AUGUST 30, 2010

At tonight's team meeting, we reviewed the Developmental Model, as we try to do every six weeks. Ben blew away Stage 3! *Yes!* Our goals are sustained eye contact for seven seconds or more, appropriate eye contact while listening to others, and central variations within his own activities. New enzymes, which help Ben to digest the food he eats and get more nutrients into his system, along with our team's incredible love and devotion, both inside and outside the playroom, have created real changes in Ben over the past two to three weeks.

Things are getting better.

God bless you, BenBen.

MONDAY, SEPTEMBER 6, 2010

One of the things profoundly missing in Ben when we started our Son-Rise Program was interest in other people. Ben never asked questions about others, never seemed to care what other people were feeling, never looked at people (of course), and never showed any interest in the experiences or activities of others.

During this past weekend visiting Sean's parents in Rhode Island, however, as we went through a drive-through to get Sean some coffee, Ben saw where we were and asked, "Daddy, are you hungry?" For a normal child, a commonplace inquiry. For a child with autism, an amazing question! Sean and I looked at each other with saucer eyes and grinned. I almost yelped.

Then, while Ben was in the bathtub later that weekend, Sean commented that one of the bath toys, a certain Michael the Frog, was missing. Ben yelled out in response, "Oh no! That's Alina's favorite frog! She's going to be so upset!"

Finally, one recent afternoon, I was whining about the fact that I had left a book I was reading at the airport. In response, Ben immediately exclaimed, "Mommy, we should go back to the airport to find your book!"

Another big problem for Ben has been a lack of expressiveness in his language. But Ben is getting more creative and enthusiastic in his communication all the time. When we were about to leave to come home from Rhode Island, for example, Ben looked up at me in the middle of the snack he was eating and exclaimed, spontaneously and with marked enthusiasm, "I am so excited to be going home!" This expression was noteworthy not only because it was a contextually appropriate and enthusiastic exclamation of a feeling he was having at that moment, but also because he interrupted his eating—an intense sensory experience for Ben, and one that he does not often choose to interrupt with deliberate, spontaneous verbal communication—to tell me what he was feeling.

Then, later, as we were on the trip home and Sean and I were talking about the weekend, I couldn't remember exactly what Ben had said he was excited about, so I asked Ben, "Honey, what did you tell me you were excited about?" and Ben responded, smiling, "About going home, Mommy!"

In the past, when we have gone to Rhode Island, Ben has had a very hard time handling the stimulation of being in a new environment, sleeping in a new bed, and having lots of new people around, even people he already knows, like his grandparents. But this weekend, he seemed to have no trouble at all.

Ben played with Alina and their eleven-year-old cousin, Becca. He even created a game to plan a surprise for Grandma Ro, which was to put lots of stuffed animals on her rocking chair. The game was a total hit with everyone. I'm not sure how controlling Ben was during the game. Ben tends to order his peers about, which is still symptomatic of the autism, trying to create security in an insecure situation (*i.e.*, playing with other children). Regardless, everyone had fun.

The only meltdown took place when I decided to go home on Sunday instead of Monday, because it was raining and we couldn't go to the beach, and I was concerned that being indoors all day would not go well. Ben was having so much fun that he didn't want to leave a day early, and he shed some tears. But it all passed in fifteen-plus minutes. Afterwards, Grandma Ro asked, "Does he always let go that easily?" Um . . .

WEDNESDAY, SEPTEMBER 8, 2010

At nigh-nighs tonight, I commented to the children that Ben's plantar wart has not gone away yet. Alina said, "It's still there because Ben has autism." I said, "No, autism is in the brain and warts are on the feet, so they have nothing to do with one another."* Whenever Alina mentions autism in Ben's presence, I feel uneasy because I have never taken the time to think through whether or not to talk to Ben about the fact that he has autism. I paused for a moment, thinking about the issue and my lack of clarity.

---

* Actually Alina's comment was more accurate than it sounds, in my opinion, since Ben's possibly compromised immune system may be more susceptible to viruses, the likes of which cause plantar warts!

Suddenly Ben broke the silence, saying quietly, "I know another word for autism. It's Son-Rise. Or it's also my playroom." This was the first time I have ever heard Ben use the word *autism*. I replied, "Yes, Ben, your Son-Rise Program is for your autism. When you are all done with autism, you will graduate from your Son-Rise Program. And then you will be able to go to school—if you want to—and without the autism you will feel much more comfortable with other people!"

I then experienced some fear that Ben would hear judgment in my words, as if I had suggested that his autism is a bad thing we need to get rid of. But of course I have no real idea what Ben was thinking at that moment. Actually, I'm quite certain he was probably thinking about rabbits on the ceiling or something along those lines. In any case, Ben then responded, "My playroom—homeschool—is for autism." I replied, "Yes, Ben, and you are such a smart boy to understand that!"

Who knew? I surely didn't. My son knows he has autism and that's why we do homeschool—*i.e.*, his Son-Rise Program—in his Son-Rise Program playroom.

He doesn't miss much.

THURSDAY, SEPTEMBER 9, 2010

Ben and I were coming up the stairs from homeschool today so Ben could go potty. He wanted me to put his T-ball set into his room. I promised him I would, but only if he promised to go right back down to homeschool after he went potty.

Ben replied, "I will, because I know homeschool is important for me."

I asked, "Why is homeschool important for you, honey?"

He answered, "Because sometimes I get afraid to make friends."

SATURDAY, SEPTEMBER 11, 2010

So now we have been on Enzymedica's SpectrumGold for three days. It is an enzyme compound that helps to digest gluten, casein, lactose, phenols, and some other stuff, but those are the main ones.

As I wrote last night, Ben has been nonresponsive for a couple of days; today he was an utter zombie. He wouldn't even look at me, ism-ing all day, both in the playroom and out, though he wanted kisses at nigh-nighs and was clearly aware of us and quite communicative at different parts of the day.

So I'm thinking, earlier today, "Okay, Sus, stay happy, love Ben, it's all part of our journey." But I'm a little thrown by the autistic behaviors and affect, which we haven't seen in a while.

Then later in the day, I was up in my office, and I decided to pick up a book about biomedicals, which I haven't reviewed in a while, to see if it contained any information about enzymes. It did, so I read a few pages. There, lo and behold, I read (with heavy paraphrasing here), "Expect die-off when you start enzymes. It may last for one to two weeks; if symptoms persist beyond two weeks, you should consider alternate approaches or perhaps just different types of enzymes."

Voila. Zombie mode (probably) explained.

I feel much better. It's logical. The fact that we are seeing die-off type symptoms also suggests that the enzymes are having an impact. So here's hoping.

MONDAY, SEPTEMBER 13, 2010

Communion

Today Ben was very autistic, and very tired.

---

* Die-off refers to the expiring of the pathogenic bacteria in the gut as new and healthy bacteria start to grow. Die-off usually creates a worsening of symptoms before improvement.

We spent thirty-five minutes circuiting the room just now, walking around the playroom, over and over and over again. Ben had no expression on his face, he kicked things around the floor, he dragged his fingers over the wall (sensory stimulation), and he made little squeaking noises from time to time. I joined Ben, circuiting, kicking things around the floor, dragging my fingers over the wall, and making little squeaking noises whenever he did. At one point I took off my socks, because Ben had bare feet, and it really changed the experience. I mirrored his actions, loving him deeply with every step, and experienced what he did, in my own way.

It was one of the most deeply connected experiences I have ever had. It was a deeply intense, restful, fun, and passionate experience of communion with my child. I was disappointed when the next person arrived to begin their session. I actually felt as though I had been meditating for several hours.

Either the enzymes are working in a good way and this is die-off, or they are working in a not-good way and we'll put the kibosh on them in a couple of weeks. But today's session, which brought me back to an experience of Ben's autism I have not had in over a year, was a gift.

Not only did it show me how far we have come in such a short time, but it also was a moment of joy for me. St. Francis said, "It is better to love than to be loved." It's even better to feel both, and I know now that Ben loves me as much as I love him. The Son-Rise Program and God have given me that.

On we go.

WEDNESDAY, SEPTEMBER 29, 2010

Ben has a fever. Fever usually makes Ben lucid, and today Ben's fever also brought on lightning-speed responsiveness. This afternoon, for example, around 4:30, upon returning home from Alina's swim lesson, I walked into Ben's room, where he was sleeping. He opened his eyes and immediately threw out, "Hi Mom." (I don't know if he has ever called me "Mom" before!) I said, "Hello, sweetheart!" A split-second later, Ben exclaimed, "I have great news!" Wow. I replied, "How exciting! I can't wait to hear it!" "Well," Ben continued, "I know how I can get well! All I have to do is sleep until seven, and I will be well!" "Fantastic!" I returned. "Have a wonderful sleep until then." I left him there, and he slept for another ninety minutes or so before coming downstairs.

Also, we have started him on magnesium capsules, which together with a new enzyme called No-Fenol, is having a wonderful effect on his elimination. We had at least three, if not four, days of no straining and well-formed poops! Ah, the things that bring me joy.

He's getting better . . . socially

A friend of ours left her toddler son, named Joe, with us today while she did some volunteer work. Ben saw the child and the mother. I told Ben the woman's name was Ellen, to which he exclaimed, "Hi Ellen." He then inquired, "How are your twin boys?" (Ellen has older twin boys, whom Ben knows, but has not seen for years.) He then showed Joe some Dr. Seuss books and was overall extremely and appropriately friendly. I was very proud of my seven-year-old.

Ben is still doing a lot of verbal ism-ing. His current obsessive focus, for example, is the set of early reader books by Dr. Seuss, which Ben refers to as the "Mr. Begin books." We are all required to name Mr. Begin books constantly, throughout the day. It's like an ice breaker for Ben in conversations. He still constantly fixates on verbal isms like this, not always to the exclusion of normal, context-appropriate conversation, but still much of the time. More often than not. I trust that will fall away as he needs it less.

TUESDAY, OCTOBER 5, 2010

Choosing love over fear

Today I hurtled downward on an emotional roller coaster.

What happened? Ben went back into a remote state, and was ism-y and nonresponsive much of the day. Poor tyke, he's still feverish and congested. He was in homeschool for a lot of hours, because he's happiest there. But he was also exerting energy being in there, and maybe tomorrow I will keep him upstairs to rest. Actually, I think I will ask him where he feels he'll get better best. He knows himself better than anyone.

But I'm not handling his autism so well right now.

The truth is I hate it. I hate seeing him ism-ing. I hate seeing him looking off into the lights on the ceiling and not telling me what he likes about them or why he's looking at them. I'm sick of joining. I want him to be responsive all the time, the way he has been on some days, and to answer my questions when I ask them, rather than seeming not to hear me and staying within himself. I don't believe he's defying me or that he's doing anything other than taking care of himself. I just feel like he's locked in this autistic world when he's ism-ing, and I want him to unlock the door and come back to me. I want him to throw his arms around me and hug me and say, "I love you, Mommy!" like I read about in a book about a mother who used enzymes to cure her autistic kids, whose sons are now expressive and affectionate and loving. I want that.

It's a tease, having him go up and down like this.

So what do my spiritual practices teach me about coping with stuff like this? My twelve-step program tells me to let go of negative thinking, stay in the day, let go and let God, and accept life on life's terms. The Son-Rise Program tells me that my beliefs are motivating me to choose unhappiness (fear) and that I can change my beliefs to change my feelings and my life. Sean tells me Ben's current ups and downs are understandable and rational, and to do what I can to identify anything we can do differently on a concrete level (*e.g.*, food, different enzymes, activities, etc.).

What's the right answer?

Gratitude and acceptance of Ben's autism. Acceptance doesn't mean I have to like the situation, just that I need to not resist it if I want peace. The Serenity Prayer tells me to do what I can do and to accept, with grace, the things I cannot change. For today, I can't change Ben's autism. For today, I can let go of what I want and practice gratitude for what is. I have Ben. He has come so far. He actually wants to be with us most of the time. We're doing lots of work to help him get better, and part of that involves detoxification, with its attendant detours into autistic behavior. Moreover, he's been sick for days on end, and ism-ing for him is probably the equivalent of holing myself off upstairs with the flat panel and watching cheesy chick flicks for a day or two. I need to cut him, and myself, some slack.

SATURDAY, OCTOBER 9, 2010

Choosing happiness when Ben chooses unhappiness

A year and a half ago, Alina turned four, and we had a big princess party for her. My friend, Sharon, who does these princess parties, came and transformed our loft into a magical princess palace. A dozen or so children attended the party, boys and girls. The boys were pirates, and the girls were princesses. Ben, six at the time, wanted nothing to do with Alina's party and announced he would have his own party two floors down in the children's activities room. We assumed that the boys would want to be away from the girly princess stuff and that they would stay downstairs with Ben.

The party came off brilliantly, but not for Ben. As it turned out, none of the boys wanted to be downstairs with him. Understandably, they wanted to be upstairs where the action was, that is, with Princess Sharon in the loft. Ben was heartily, painfully disappointed and cried for the duration of the party. When I came downstairs and saw Ben sobbing, my heart broke. I made a decision to enjoy Alina's party anyway. It was her day, and I didn't want it to be spoiled because her brother was feeling sorry for himself. I succeeded in putting my focus on Alina for the rest of the day and let Sean take care of Ben. It turned out okay, but I found it painful to see Ben so unhappy. I hadn't yet learned the wisdom of choosing personal happiness regardless of your children's choosing happiness or not.

This evening I had a flashback to that party. We had plans to spend the evening with friends of ours to listen to Son-Rise Program parenting CDs and discuss how those principles apply to our own parenting challenges. Our friends' babysitting fell through, and because I really wanted to get together with our friends, I offered to have their three children come to our house and have our babysitter watch all five of the kids.

It was not a well thought-out decision, and I didn't consult Sean. It was not a structured, Son-Rise Program-based playdate, where Ben would be taken care of and in control. It was a good, though hard, lesson for me.

Now our children know these children quite well; they think of them as cousins. There is a daughter who is Ben's age, and twins who are Alina's age. They are very sweet, neurotypical children. Ben was excited all day about their coming. When they arrived, he became *manically* excited. After a little while, Sean and I became concerned, because the visiting children were ignoring Ben. I spoke with my friend, the mother, and we discussed the best approach to help the children all get along. It was a rather awkward conversation, because it was a little late to be prepping the children.

Suddenly, the children started a game of running races. Ben was completely involved and participating. The older child was uninterested; it was a childish game, and she is extremely precocious. But the four other children had a blast. I actually videotaped it. I remarked to our friends that this was God's way of saying, "Chill out, Sean and Susan!" Ben was clearly having a great time and connecting beautifully.

A little later, the adults adjourned to the loft for food and discussion, while the children remained below with their dinners and television on the evening's itinerary. About twenty-five minutes later, however, Sean interrupted our discussion to remark, "I don't hear the television. I'm going to see what's going on."

He returned several minutes later, announcing, "It has not gone well at all. Ben is alone in his room having a picnic with his stuffed animals. I'm going to go be with him." I sat there, feeling stunned and disappointed. I thought it had been going so well, but things had clearly gone off the tracks.

I tried to focus on the CD we were listening to but was completely distracted by thoughts of Ben and anxiety about what was happening for him downstairs. I didn't want to be away from him; I was his mother, after all. I excused myself and went downstairs.

I went to Ben's room, and found him and Sean sitting on the floor with, as noted, a picnic with stuffed animals. Ben was sobbing. I learned moments later that when the children had gone to watch television, Ben did not want them to watch television; he wanted them to play a game with him. When they declined, he went off the emotional deep end. Significantly, Ben had not eaten his dinner. Hunger has a strong impact on him and often renders him inflexible, overly sensitive, and emotional.

I told Sean I wanted to be with Ben, and he returned to our guests, where they spent the next forty-five minutes or so enjoying each other's company. I, on the other hand, tried to love and be with Ben. He cried pretty much the entire time. He denied, also, that he was sad and asserted, repeatedly and emphatically, "I'm always happy! I'm never sad! These are tears because I'm cold, not because I'm sad!"

He then spilled a cup of water on the picnic blanket (his Pooh blanket) and decided to go downstairs again. But when we went downstairs, it got worse, because he heard the television and cried even harder. I tried to stay happy but eventually ended up crying myself. *I forgot that I could be happy despite Ben's choice to be unhappy.*

Ben wrote down the word "CRY" on a piece of paper and told me to bring it to Alina because he wanted her to be disappointed the way he was. Aha! So he was disappointed. I asked him how come he was disappointed, and he said, "I won't tell you!" He just refused to talk about it.

Somehow he has decided that being upset is unacceptable, that he is "always happy," and that he will not discuss details of situations that upset him, regardless of how unhappy he feels. I do not like this for him; I want him to feel comfortable discussing his unhappiness or any so-called negative feelings so that he can process them in a healthy way.

In any case, when he refused to tell me why he was disappointed and became agitated and cried again, I started crying. When he saw me crying, he was taken aback, and he changed a little. He was clearly aware I was responding to his upset with my own unhappiness, and he clearly found this troubling.

Finally, the show ended, Sean and our friends came downstairs, and we got everyone ready to go. The evening ended okay, in that we read stories, did prayers, and sang songs, and a very exhausted BenBen fell asleep. He also ate a good amount of food as the guests were leaving, which immediately helped.

My lessons:
- Choose happiness regardless of Ben's choices for himself.
- Don't be so upset by Ben's disappointments. He will go through many, and it's part of being human.
- Look at all of the progress! He talked about his feelings. He wanted to be with the other children. He had half of the visit really having fun. He gave a lot of eye contact and was very interactive and responsive for much of the time.
- I realized yet again that I am still too afraid of Ben's being unhappy.
- Ben is doing great, and so are we. We're all learning.

SATURDAY, OCTOBER 30, 2010

Shared parenting: helping each other keep perspective

Ben and I had a fight about medicine today. I didn't get him to take it, but the process was great. In Sean's words, "What I loved about tonight was what Ben didn't do. Susan wanted Ben to take some medicine, and Ben adamantly refused. But,
- Ben never began to cry;
- he didn't run to his room (although he did say that he would leave the room in which he was reading if Susan tried to come in with the medicine);
- he didn't shift to an ism; and
- he didn't throw a tantrum.

"In fact, he barely raised his voice. Instead, he just talked! There were at least ten loops back and forth between Susan and Ben, with Ben firmly explaining that he was not going to take any medicine, even if it meant never having another flash (time at the computer), and even if it meant never being with Susan ever again (lol). Every statement he made was intelligent, on topic, and in a reasonable tone of voice.

"One other thing. We are trying to teach Ben to have an interest and understanding in others. Susan asked Ben if he trusted her (about the medicine), and he said he didn't. In the past, such a thought as 'trust' would have gone right by him, and he almost surely would not have responded. Instead, he said no, and further said nothing would change his mind. (Which makes sense, because he knew it was a new something or other that he didn't want to take.) That alone is tremendous!

"Think about that . . . an autistic child, talking about medicine he did not want to take, having a calm, thoughtful discussion about why he didn't want to take it, and explaining how he felt about it and his mother. It's a loving, nourishing picture I intend to hold on to."

WEDNESDAY, NOVEMBER 3, 2010

Today is Ben's eighth birthday, and it was a day filled with joy, love, and friendship. This morning Ben opened his door to a poster-board sign reading, "Happy Birthday, Ben!" He loved it. Next, Ben came downstairs where I invited him into his "Birthday Kitchen." He entered the kitchen and was met with a Wubbzy birthday to end all Wubbzy birthdays. Purple streamers (purple is Ben's favorite color) connected multiple balloons bearing images of Wubbzy, craftily designed by our beloved Oscar with marker, paper, and tape. Mylar Happy Birthday balloons adorned the walls. Ben was thrilled and smiled that huge Ben grin. It really meant a lot to him, and you could see how connected he was to the experience and what had been created for him with such love and caring by his close and extended family.

Later, during homeschool, I gave Ben one of his presents: a talking cash register. To cut to the chase, Ben actually played the game in the traditional way. He assigned one of his plastic animals, Milly the Monkey, to serve as shopkeeper. One by one, all of Mr. Bondea's animals (Mr. Bondea is Ben's fictional animal-owner in homeschool) came to the store and bought plastic foods, which Ben "sold" to the animals by typing numbers into the cash register, telling the "customers" how much it cost, and running the debit card (which came with the cash register) through the register. Ben did not: chew on the coins, ignore the game, ignore me, or bang away endlessly on the keys of the register. He also stayed with the game for at least twenty minutes. I was delighted.

Then tonight was Ben's birthday party. After opening each of the presents stacked in a pile on the kitchen table, he turned and, unsolicited by Mommy or Daddy, thanked each person graciously for their gift. He asked us repeatedly, "Is this one for me, too?"

Ben, Alina, and I made those beeswax candles for his cake, by the way. That was another big deal, a testament to Ben's fine-motor development and, more importantly, his ability to interact in a game with specific instructions. Ben actually pinched wicks into and rolled six or seven beeswax candles with me in homeschool, in preparation for his party!

A wonderful birthday.

WEDNESDAY, NOVEMBER 3, 2010

Ben just started crying hard about ten minutes ago. I ran up, and he was sitting upright in bed, more than half asleep. He calmed down while I held him, stroked his hair, and sat with him in the dark. But he continued to whimper in a series of four short moans. It was almost as if he was listening to himself making the sounds, fascinating himself by how he was emoting.

I tried to hold him, but he pulled away. I felt that familiar feeling of wanting more. I tried to stroke him, but he jerked his arm away. He is, at times, acutely sensitive to sensory experiences (other times not aware at all). Sometimes the sensory experience seems to be too much for him, like how he has to fully undress himself in order to poop.

I had that feeling that I never have with Alina, that I don't know how to comfort him and what he needs, or how to mother him. So I can pray to God to love him the best way I can, without judgment or fear, just all love and a desire to serve and care for my child.

By the way, I need to comment on my beautiful, magnificent, force-of-nature daughter, Alina. She is becoming more gentle, thoughtful, giving and generous, trusting, and happy. She amazes me in her love, passion, beauty, brilliance (both intellectual and spiritual), and creativity. She is so independent and so herself. I admire her and love her, and sometimes feel like I will burst with pride when I watch her. She is, without question, one of the world's and God's finest and most adorable creations—ever.

SUNDAY, NOVEMBER 7, 2010

Ben was again, today, incredibly interactive and responsive, with amazing, unsolicited eye contact. He was also very inflexible, but in a totally eight-year-old, "I want my way!" way.

MONDAY, NOVEMBER 15, 2010

This morning, Ben, Alina, and I were playing a game. At one point, for some reason, Alina got upset and ran out of the room crying. Ben paused, looked at me, and asked, "Mommy, why is Alina sad?"

We need a new set of rules. Sean and I are realizing that we now need to treat Ben more like a neurotypical eight-year-old and not let him get his way so much, get to be first all the time, etc. We have been so overjoyed just to have him interested in connecting with us, or in playing a game, that he has had carte blanche to get anything he wants. We have known this to be unfair to Alina, but we felt because of Ben's autism that's the way we've needed to be to make this world of human beings digestible and appealing to him. We have explained this to Alina, and she understands—somewhat.

But now, Ben is more in our world, and the rules have to change. He can't get his way all the time anymore. He has to learn that social rules apply if he wants to build friendships, including with his sister. It's challenging for us as parents, because we are used to giving Ben control. But now we have to trust that his unhappiness will not equal resumption of autism. Alina can be a tantruming tyrant and cries constantly to get what she wants. I am learning to stay comfortable and firm even in the face of her tears and rages. Now I get to be as unattached to Ben's unhappiness as I have learned—am learning to be—with Alina's unhappiness.

A note from Sean
"Two of Ben's medications are designed to improve his mitochondrial functioning, which refers to the ability of Ben's cells to convert food into energy. Since being on the medicine—almost a month now—the changes are startling, even to us. His energy has improved, his eye contact is significantly better, and we have many more normal conversations.

"Unfortunately, a side effect is some insomnia. So, last night I slept in the loft because Susan wasn't feeling well, and I didn't want to disturb her if I snored. At 4:00 AM, I heard Ben get up, so I went to his room. As soon as I walked in, he looked up and smiled at me and said, 'I wondered where you were. Mommy said you were upstairs in the loft.' I mean, to have an autistic child look up, smile, and initiate a conversation is simply incredible. It put a huge smile on my face."

FRIDAY, NOVEMBER 19, 2010

For the first time ever, Ben has begun to use colloquialisms. This is a spontaneous and unsolicited development for him. We have neither presented nor encouraged use of more casual language. He has just picked up on it, and what is especially noteworthy, what he has picked up on is not the words themselves—which he often reinvents or mis- uses—but the idea that more casual language or idiomatic language is socially "cool" and worth doing. For example, today and yesterday he used, probably no less than ten to fifteen times, the phrase, "By the way . . ." "By the way, each of my songs is similar to another song." "By the way, I finished my dinner." "By the way, Alina was the one who broke it."

Last week, he started using the word "dummer" over and over. As in, "Oh, dummer!" and "That's so dummer!" I think it was his linguistic adaptation of "Oh, crap!" or "That's so lame!" Again, what excites me is not the specific words themselves, but Ben's ap- parent newfound grasp of the value of colloquialisms in language and conceivably—though it may or may not be relevant in his mind—in social dynamics with others.

TUESDAY, NOVEMBER 30, 2010

This morning, Ben woke up at 4:30 AM. Sean went into his room, to find Ben cleaning. Sean asked Ben, "What are you doing, Ben?" Ben answered, "I'm cleaning my room, to make Mommy happy."

Ten minutes later, I invited Ben and Alina (who was by now also awake—and cleaning her room, to be like Ben!) to come snuggle with me in our bed. Alina came running, and only minutes later, Ben jumped in with us. The three of us snuggled for at least ten minutes.

I felt like the luckiest mommy in the whole world!

THURSDAY, DECEMBER 2, 2010

Ben has awakened somehow, lately, from an autistic-but-loving and ever-more-interactive child, into someone who appears more and more each day like a quirky (and forgive me, darling, but dorky) eight-year-old with odd and obsessive ways. If autism were defined solely as an isolative and exclusive condition, where there is a distinct lack of interest in others, then Ben would not currently have that label. Autism has a lot of other symptoms, of course, but its basic symptom, that a child chooses isolation rather than interaction, is almost entirely absent from Ben these days.

He is still, however, very impaired. His obsessions with random preferred topics (from specific songs to trains to Pooh to beanie babies to plastic animals to Wubbzy to Amanda Pig to his current focus—children's songs written by a fictitious composer Ben created, named "Tabafalooka") dominate his discourse and activities.

And, Ben still demonstrates additional symptoms of a problematic neurological, biochemical, and immunological condition, such as poor muscle tone, speech problems ("th" is still "f"), constant fatigue, picky eating, visual problems, and others.

Ben is a butterfly emerging from his cocoon, who is only partway emerged. He's not in full flight yet, but rather still gingerly poking holes in the chrysalis, moving tentatively and gingerly with new wings, lest he come forth too soon, unprepared.

I asked Ben, for example, on Tuesday (two days ago), if he thought he would want to go to school at some point. He said, with a twinkle, "That's ridiculous! I go to homeschool!"

I replied, "Of course you do, now, but in time, would you like to go to a school outside of home, like Alina, where big kids go?"

There was a pause and then, softly, "Yes." And then, "But not today."

THURSDAY, DECEMBER 2, 2010 (2)

Today in the playroom, I brought Ben some new bread I had made. He took two bites and said, "This tastes different. I don't want it." I asked him what it tasted like, and he replied, "Like dirt." Okay, so I'm no Betty Crocker, but dirt? So then at dinner, I presented it with less enzyme powder in it, hoping that was the problem with the earlier batch, and again, he didn't like it. Seeing it lying there on his plate, I asked him, "What do you think of the bread?" He replied, "It's terrible."

Really?

Now I don't know if I can convey this, but when he said, "It's terrible," it was different from his normal way of speaking. It was emphatic, which is normal for Ben, but there was an appropriateness to the language he chose and a deliberate casualness about it that felt both commonplace and nonautistic.

Later, Alina came in, and I gave her a piece of the new bread. She tried it and said, "It's a little good." I asked, "Not very good?" She replied, "No, not very good." Ben then interjected, looking right in my eyes, "That's what I was talking about!" For Ben to make such a comment was amazing. Inconceivable. Yet here it was, and here *he* is, changing and using language that is contextually appropriate and joining us, totally unsolicited, in conversation.

He's changing. He's more interactive, aware, and interested in others. At the toy store last weekend, he asked if he could buy an Angelina Ballerina book for Alina for Hanukkah, then asked the store clerk (at my suggestion), "if you would please wrap this present for my sister, Alina." Then last night, for Hanukkah, he and Alina spent almost an hour playing with their first-night, joint present, a science-experiment set.

So what's doing it?

I think it's the mitochondrial supports, specifically CoQ10 and carnitine, because that's when these observable changes began. He's also been on the SCD yogurt for two weeks, and we're up to half a teaspoon/day, with no problematic behaviors like when we tried the yogurt a few months ago. Ben's also back, for two weeks at least, on fish oil, and we're up to 5 ml of that a day. We're doing the epsom salts cream on his legs, arms, and tummy every night, consistently. Ben will have a glutathione shot on Saturday (Sean's driving him down and back, six hours in the car, for a ten-minute appointment for his shot. What won't we do for the people we love?). The biomedical interventions are clearly helping.

But the most significant factor, in my opinion? *Ben wants to be with us.* He wants to be himself, with us, and connected.

FRIDAY, DECEMBER 10, 2010

Shockingly, I take Ben's miracles for granted these days. There are so many examples.

- I ask Ben a question, and he answers so often now that I am slightly taken aback if he doesn't answer. I now think to myself, "How come he's not answering?" instead of "Of course he's not answering." In the past, Ben never responded to questions; he actually only started doing so four or five months ago.
- Sean and I are having frequent conversations about Ben going to school this fall.

- Ben looks at me, right in the eyes, both while listening and while talking, constantly. More often than not.
- Ben communicates lovingly and expressively about how he feels and often asks others how they feel about particular things.
- Ben often tries to help Alina with problems she's having.
- Ben often tells us when he's tired, rather than just lying down on the floor in random (and often inappropriate) places.
- Ben is willing to take turns.
- Ben is often willing to play by the rules of new games, even regular board games like children's Monopoly.
- Ben makes phone calls to people now.
- Ben knows his home address and phone number now!
- Ben is reading at a third-grade level (he should be in second grade) and does math at a first-grade level—this from the boy who has had no formal schooling of any kind nor any math or reading training at home in two years!
- Ben is constantly affectionate, abundant with hugs, kisses, and vehement demands for my attention, such as "Mommy, I want you now!" and "Mommy, eyes on me!"
- My son and I sit, some mornings, and make music together. I play the piano, and we both sing. Tabafalooka songs. It is heaven for me. Singing with Ben and snuggling some nights with Alina are my current moments of joy.
- Most significantly, Ben constantly chooses to be part of our world now, and not only in the larger sense of part of the earth's community of human beings. He is also part of our family now, interacting meaningfully on a consistent basis, often delightfully, almost always whimsically, in his unique, brilliant, gorgeous, musical, quirky, endlessly imaginative ways.

Sean notes that Ben still doesn't say, "I love you." I observe frequent language retrieval problems, which interrupt his social interactions. He still speaks in a super-high voice. He still poops in his birthday suit. He is still obsessed with verbal isms.

But I am patient. I love this journey. As Ben grows, we grow, and as we grow, Ben grows. I don't care how long it takes. I enjoy the moments.

TUESDAY, DECEMBER 14, 2010

Right now, Ben is rigid, controlling, histrionic, completely focused, in love with Mommy (which I adore), all rigid gaming in the playroom, very interactive, great eye contact, friendly, and fun. Regarding word retrieval, Ben remains greatly impaired. I noticed it especially today when Ben wanted to tell an older friend of his, Sam, about a guinea pig he made up. Ben said to Sam, "Oh I forgot, I have something to tell you!" Sam replied, "What was that, Ben?" Ben said, "I had a guinea pig—I mean—er—it was a—um" and then he got stuck and couldn't go on. Sam was incredible and said, "Oh wow, Ben, that's cool!" But Ben was clearly frustrated at his own inability to get his words out.

SATURDAY, DECEMBER 25, 2010

Our current focus in Ben's Son-Rise Program playroom is on flexibility and inspiring Ben to play games that we initiate as well as ones he chooses for himself. We also want to develop Ben's interest in others and continue to encourage him to find fun in other people's interests and experiences, rather than just in his own.

FRIDAY, JANUARY 7, 2011

This evening, I watched as Sean was reading *Pinkalicious* to the children, and Ben leaned his whole body against his daddy, his head on

Sean's shoulder, and relaxed—like any other little boy in love with his daddy would do.

Our team goal for the next two weeks:

We will inspire Ben to be interested in *us*! By bringing in themes about things we're interested in and sharing information about ourselves and focusing on ourselves, we will inspire Ben to be excited about other people. This will greatly help him build the social muscles he needs to be successful in peer relationships, and in the upcoming playdates I plan to schedule for him.

THURSDAY, JANUARY 13, 2011

Sea of changes

The phrase "sea change" comes from Shakespeare's *The Tempest.*[*] We are, as a family, in a sea of changes, even as we witness a sea change in Ben. And our life is at once both rich and endlessly strange.

Alina is moving through her second half of kindergarten, transforming into a reader, and ever more intense. She grows even more plastic-faced as her moods and desires shift with untamable suddenness, from Jekyll to Hyde and then back to Jekyll. Alina is intense; from sheer sweetness and radiant, sunshiny delight to boiling rage and crocodile tears, volcanic and demanding. Then back to sunshine. She is something to watch. A *true* tempest, or a night sky, with a whole month of weather patterns speeded up to mere moments.

---

[*] Full fathom five thy father lies;
Of his bones are coral made;
Those are pearls that were his eyes:
Nothing of him that doth fade
But doth suffer a sea-change
Into something rich and strange.
(1.2.396-401), Ariel

Then Sean and I, who continue on our journeys of partnership, parenting, and self-discovery. We're doing well, observing each other's reactions, affirming and celebrating the strengths, and gently chiding each other on our weak moments.

Then Ben, who is a sea change in motion. He no longer resembles the autistic child he was even a year ago. Now he is connected, part of us. He is expressive and emotional and passionate. Tonight he actually made himself cry in telling a story he made up about a little blue squirrel who was rejected by his little brown mates and deeply lonely. The story had a happy ending, with a little lonely boy finding the lonely blue squirrel and the two of them living happily ever after, but Ben literally shed tears as he told the story! (I told him he was going to be a great method actor.)

Ben is finding his place among other people, children and adults. He's aware. His internal switch has flipped, the lights are on, the energy is coursing through him, and the connection is electric—especially for those of us who were with him before the lights came on.

MONDAY, JANUARY 31, 2011

I love you too!

Every night, for years, when I kissed Ben goodnight, I always said, "I love you, and I am so proud of you." Ben never said "I love you" back, though he has told me he loves me several times. Sometimes he said, "Thanks" (which comes out "Sanks," since Ben still can't do his th's). I know he loves me. But I have always wished he would say the words.

Then last night, I said, as I always do, "Goodnight, Ben, I love you. And I'm so proud of you." Ben replied, "Sanks." Then he paused, seemed to realize something, looked at me, and said, "And I love you too!"

TUESDAY, FEBRUARY 1, 2011

I love you too, Daddy's turn

This morning, Ben said, "I love you too!" to Sean, as Sean was leaving for a business trip to Philadelphia. This is only the second time Ben has ever said I love you to Sean, the first time being just a few weeks ago. What do we make of that? Not sure, but Sean was over the moon.

A substantive conversation with Ben about school

Today Alina, Ben, and I were in the playroom talking about pets. Ben would like a kitten, and Alina and I would like a puppy—or two. I told the children that once Ben and Alina were both in school for a full year, we could get our pets. For real.

A few minutes later, Ben asked, "How many more days of home-school do I have, Mommy?" Taken aback by his question, I replied, "Well, that depends on whether you want to go to school this fall or not, sweetheart." Three seconds passed, and Ben responded, "I would." My heart skipped a beat. This is the first time Ben has expressed a preference for going to school. I replied, "Well, in that case, you have a lot of days, about 200 or more until the fall comes and school will start."

Then Ben asked, "What grade would I be in, Mommy?" Again, the heart skipping beats. "Well, BenBen, to be honest, Daddy and I don't really know what grade you would be in. Because with reading and math, you are at a fourth and second grade level. But with being with other kids and making friends, you are just starting out, probably first grade. So we don't know. What grade would you like to be in?"

Ben answered, "I don't know." So I asked, "Would you like to be in Alina's class? She's in first grade." Ben made a slight face. (I would call it a grimace, but Ben doesn't grimace. He just pauses and frowns slightly). Then he stated, firmly, "I would not want to be in Alina's class."

"Really honey?" I asked. "Then maybe you would want to be with other eight-year-olds?"

"Yes."

"Well," I continued, "that is why we are doing more playdates. So you can practice being with friends and learning how to be with other children your age."

Ben said, "But I have friends! Like Sam and Charlie!"

"Yes," I replied, "but in school you will be in a group of children, and you will need to learn to be comfortable in a group. Do you think you would be comfortable in a group now?"

"Yes," Ben said. "I would."

Then Ben went over and picked out a small, plastic panda and began telling me a story about the little panda who was afraid to go to school because he didn't know anybody. Suddenly he interrupted his story and ran over to me and put his arms around me.

"Mommy," he cried, "what if I get scared and don't know the other eight-year-olds?"

"Well, BenBen, then you will get to know them and be friends with them," I replied.

"Yes," said Ben. "I can introduce . . ."

"Yes, honey?" I said.

". . . myself," finished Ben.

"Absolutely. And what do you think they will say to you when you introduce yourself?"

"They will say, 'Hello, Ben, my name is blahblahblah!'"

"Exactly!" I practically yelled.

I was stunned. My son expressed a desire to go to school with other children (pet motivated or not, it's still wonderful). Then he articulated his fears and was open to a strategy for working through them.

Ben's progress is tremendous and irrefutable, but he still has a lot of autism. I see it in his obsessive focus on his special interests, namely storytelling about characters he makes up, and rigid fixations on certain toys, books, and songs. These obsessions universally permeate Ben's experiences, and he uses them to navigate his way through the world. In other words, though he is willing to play our games, he always returns to his obsessive interests. Yet every day he is more expressive, present, flexible, and connected to people.

So I don't really know where Ben is right now. Sometimes I feel very confused. Is Ben ready to step out into the world? How will Ben interact with neurotypical children? Is he ready for eight-year-olds in school, or should we hold him back a grade or two?

It's hard to be unclear. There are always so many issues I still face: constant feelings of inadequacy, fears of my own incompetency, and frustration with my lack of understanding. What sustains and strengthens me, always, is gratitude. Gratitude feeds both my acceptance and my faith, and enables me to keep going forward, showing up for my children and my marriage. I talk to others about my gratitude, and I focus mentally on my blessings. I have more blessings than troubles, when I list them all out.

Most of all, I am grateful to be on the journey with my family. We're all kind of messed up, in certain ways, each of us complicated and difficult. But I understand more than I used to how to love my family and how to be with my children, especially. Sean and I are compatible, similar in the ways that count. But the children? I have had to learn how to be with them, and it's been hard. To be a Son-Rise Program parent, I had to become lighter, more silly, less cerebral, and more in the moment. I had to learn how to *play*, which was terribly hard for me. In doing so, however, I learned how to be with my children, and with any other children. I understand now that play is as serious a matter for children as work and relationships are for adults. Play defines their world. I understand this now, so I can be with my children in a way that meets them where they are. I can truly, actually, *be with them.*

Chapter 4
Struggling to Connect

"*Fluffer just loves meatloaf! It's one of the treats his favorite student, A. M., always gives him when she gets to take him home for the weekend. 'Aw, Fluffer, you're so cute!' said A.M. 'Would you like some more meatloaf?'*"

Suddenly, one of the other students interrupted, exclaiming, "Ben, you're boring!" Undeterred, Ben continued with his story. "We're going to the park this afternoon, Fluffer! I can't wait to show you the fountain there!' said A.M." The classmate interrupted a second time, repeating emphatically, "Ben, we don't want to hear your stories! They're boring!"

This time, Ben stopped. He paused and asked, "Why not?" The boy answered, "Because we don't want to hear about stories, or people. We want to do stuff!" Ben's face fell. He stayed quiet for the rest of the class.

BEN PREPARES FOR SCHOOL

The next chapter of Ben's recovery began in the fall of 2011, when Ben began academic homeschooling, and we transitioned into a part-time Son-Rise Program. This period lasted until September 2012, when we moved to New York. After almost three years of a full-time Son-Rise Program, Ben had progressed enough for me to begin an actual academic curriculum with him.* During this period, Ben became an active part of a group of homeschooled children, the majority of whose parents used a Waldorf curriculum.

This new stage, during which Ben experimented with and developed his first peer relationships, was an intense social-learning period for Ben. He made constant social errors and had his heart broken more than once. Perpetually, however, Ben returned to the plate. He was as invested in developing social connections for himself as we were for him. My heart bled when he stumbled, but at the same time I was acutely aware of his commitment to his own social development, and it thrilled me.

This second period was Ben's most difficult period thus far. Earlier in his life, when Ben was completely submerged in autism, he actually seemed quite happy. He was cut off from others, and, living unto himself most of the time, Ben was faced with no social risks. Accordingly, with the exception of frequent feelings of anxiety (expressed through his tantrums), he stayed mostly in a state of comfortable control. Later, during the first few years of our Son-Rise Program, I shielded him from social risks. We chose not to go on vacations, visit grandparents, spend time with friends or extended family, and go to children's events or social functions. I knew Ben wasn't ready, and I made his recovery my top priority. He was, as we learned at our courses, "cooking" in the playroom, and I wanted him cooking at top speed!

During these early years, Ben had almost no exposure to peers. Even in the third year when Ben started to have playdates, I held them in his playroom, where he retained a substantial sense of control. I also deliberately kept his interactions brief (no more than thirty to

---

* In our home, we referred to Ben's Son-Rise Program as "homeschool," as an easy vernacular for us. It was entirely Son-Rise Program work, however, with no academic content.

sixty minutes) to minimize the amount of stimulation Ben faced as he gingerly began to move forward into more contact with his peers. By fall 2011, however, at the start of our fourth year of Ben's Son-Rise Program, he had emerged substantially from autism, and we were able to transition him into a part-time program. Part-time meant, for us, an average of ten to twelve hours weekly in the playroom instead of twenty-five to thirty-five. Once he began his part-time program, Ben had many more social opportunities. Significantly, over this period, he developed a desperate desire to be with other children and in school. As an active participant in our homeschooling group, Ben had tremendous opportunity for interactions with peers, learning experiences, and emotional exposure. New to the game, he was extremely vulnerable. Through these interactions, Ben began to recognize more and more the differences between himself and other children, especially between himself and other boys his age. Ben told me once, after he emerged from autism, that before his Son-Rise Program, he always felt "on the outside of things." His desire to be *on the inside* dominated this second period of our Son-Rise Program journey.

Additionally, during most of this second stage, I had not yet discovered the Body Ecology Diet (BED), which ultimately turned out to be the most effective diet for Ben. Accordingly, Ben was still having major problems with digestion and, consequently, with energy and functioning. In light of these ongoing biomedical challenges, in conjunction with his utter lack of social experience, Ben's first connections with peers were extremely problematic. By this point, he wanted friends more than anything in the world, but he frequently misinterpreted social cues, and the results were often catastrophic. His mistakes crushed him and us as well as we watched him stumble forward. At such times, out of sheer self-preservation, I compared Ben to where he had been before his Son-Rise Program, rather than to some vision of perfect recovery that would inevitably depress me. We grew personally during this period, but it was not without cost.

BLOGGING AS BEN PREPARES FOR SCHOOL

Note: These postings begin in 2011. Ben is eight years old and has just completed his first round of IVIG, an aggressive treatment for an autoimmune disorder with which Ben had been diagnosed. It is four days after our conversation about his wanting to go to school.*

SATURDAY, FEBRUARY 5, 2011

We're not out of the woods yet. Today I went with the children to their gymnastics classes. Ben does Special Olympics at the same studio where Alina takes her gymnastics class, which works out great. I watched both children for almost forty-five minutes.

I observed several things. I watched Ben stare off into space in a characteristically autistic manner. I saw him sing the endless children's songs that are his predominant ism these days. After the class, I saw him trying to tell his coach that she should keep on doing her gymnastics practices—but stumble on the words and tell her to keep practicing her drumming instead. Later I listened as he came to me and explained how he had meant to say one thing but said another instead. He's aware of his stumblings, though he doesn't seem to judge himself.

On the other hand, I also saw a child full of excitement and happiness at being with the other children and his coaches, following

---

* IVIG stands for intravenous immunoglobulin and is a process whereby the plasma of other people is infused into a patient, whose own plasma contains antibodies that are creating an autoimmune reaction in the patient's body. PANDAS stands for Pediatric Autoimmune Neurologic Disorder Associated with Strep and is a clinical diagnosis with symptoms of anxiety, obsessive-compulsive disorder, and aggression. Ben's doctor had given him a PANDAS diagnosis due to his obsessiveness and his anxiety and recommended IVIG for treatment.

all the instructions, doing the exercises, and having a ball. He was polite, friendly, sweet, and observant.

Just not out of the woods yet.

He's made progress, is loving and expressive, and mauls us with hugs and kisses constantly. Today I showed him my Facebook profile picture, which is a picture of him and me. As soon as he saw it, he cried out, "I'm so happy you have a picture of you and me there!" Then he grabbed me around the neck with his arms and kissed me really hard.

He's more responsive, energetic, articulate, and aware of others. He's context-appropriate much more often.

SATURDAY, FEBRUARY 19, 2011

Feeling it from the inside

Note: Part of Ben's PANDAS syndrome is a phobia around what his doctor terms "contamination." Essentially, Ben removes all of his clothing every time he poops to avoid any possibility of his clothing getting stained. Last week I began a rewards system where I pay him to keep his clothing on. Ben seemed open to it.

On a delightful note, Ben's motivation to keep his clothing on has quickly turned away from a material reward. On Wednesday, I told Ben if he kept doing so well, I was going to run out of money, since I owed him so much by that point. Ben responded by saying, "But I'm not doing this for the money. I'm doing it because I want to be a good boy."

I was touched. I thought to myself, Ben is motivated to do the right thing because he wants to do the right thing. He isn't doing the right thing for an M&M or even for the books he wants. He just wants to please us and be good. I am so glad he is a Son-Rise Program child!

Ben is also very keen lately on the idea that he is a growing boy, "almost a grown-up, Mommy!" and that he wants to be kind. He has told us more than once that he doesn't like teasing because it's not kind, and he only wants to be kind. Ben seems to be an idealist and a believer in goodness in himself and others. Even sick (he has a stomach flu right now), he remains cheerful, engaged, animated, interactive, and flexible.

Overall, since the IVIG and the post-procedure fogginess subsided, Sean and I have both observed heightened responsiveness, heightened clarity of language, and more alertness and sensitivity to others. It's subtle and difficult to assess since we spend so much time with him, but the progress is there.

Marital struggles

Sean and I fought today. He felt discounted when I wouldn't or couldn't take in a work story he wanted very much to share with me. I was sick with nausea and fatigue, the story was complicated, and I'm poor at following the legal intricacies of his cases, though I do try to understand them. He became angry; I got defensive and then angry. We yelled and argued, in front of the children, and stayed angry and emotional for a number of hours. It was terrible.

I went to our bedroom and cried, feeling, by turns, sorry for myself, self-righteous, indignant, and confused about what I had done wrong. Sean fumed and reflected; some time later, he came to me and apologized. We discussed both of our errors and mutually apologized.

I asked the children, sitting nearby at that point, whether our fighting troubled them, and did they think we fought a lot? Alina answered, "Not really." Ben replied, "Not so much." I guess they understand that Mommy and Daddy blow off steam at each other; I guess we haven't destroyed their psyches. We'll keep working on it. Marriage, like parenting, is a journey. Now there is peace again. The children are having their TV night (once a week; two PBS shows, very exciting). Sean is exercising. I'm writing and processing my life, our life.

MONDAY, FEBRUARY 21, 2011

A perspective for all of us to consider

I asked the children last week if they knew what my perfect day was. I told them my perfect day was any day I spend with them. Alina said her perfect day was spending all day with me. Ben said, "My perfect day is every day!"

"This is the best day of my life!"

Ben had an unbelievable day today, and I am walking on air. He had a playdate with a neurotypical seven-and-a-half-year-old boy, the son of a dear friend of mine who drove up from the Cape for the playdate. Because of the long distance, they stayed for four hours.

The boys had a great time, and had so much fun playing together. Ben was engaged, engaging, responsive, polite, and loving. The little boy had a good time and said so. We did playroom time for half an hour, with a scavenger hunt theme Sean created last night. I had a blast leading the boys through the game, and they had fun, too. Then we came back upstairs and had free play, snacks, and more free play. Ben even showed his friend how to do some of his vision and core-strengthening exercises!

As we were coming upstairs after the scavenger hunt, Ben said to me, "This is the best day of my life!" I smiled. Later, Ben said to his friend, "Zander, I love you, you're so cool!" Zander grinned, laughed, and said, "Ben said he loves me, Mommy!" We explained to Zander that Ben was actually just trying to say he thought Zander was an awesome person. I don't think Zander was upset to be told that! Later, his mommy asked Zander if it was a fun playdate, and he replied, in a totally sincere way, "Yeah! It was!"

In sum

Four hours. No incident. Ben totally happy. No ism-ing afterwards. Ben was gracious, friendly, and interested in his new friend. I feel hopeful about school for Ben. He handled himself so well, and only needed reminders to respond sometimes when people asked him a question. That's the stage we're at: he has the capacity to respond, knows how to do it, and just needs to be reminded sometimes.

Ben told me what he did at school today

This evening Ben and I had dinner together, and I asked him what he did at Brain Balance today, with his teacher, Kathleen. Brain Balance is a part motor-skills, part academic-skills program designed to eliminate or at least improve the imbalanced hemispheric strength in Ben's brain. In response to my question, Ben replied, "We did math." I then asked, "Did you do addition or subtraction?" He responded, "Subtraction." Then he added, "And we have to buy presents for my teachers, because next week is the Brain Balance party for the last week of classes."

For those of you without autistic children, this is certainly uninteresting dialogue.

For those of you with autistic children, you will understand why I am crying.

Pointing a finger

Well, sometimes it's great to be me. I went in for my afternoon session with Ben just now, and God gave me such a gift. I was telling Ben about the fact that some of the people who live with us will be leaving in the next four to eight weeks. After I told him the details, I asked him how he felt about these people leaving. He paused for about five to ten seconds and seemed to grimace a little. I expected this reaction, because he loves these people dearly.

Ben replied, softly, "Happy."

Surprised, I asked him, "Happy? Why?"

Ben started, "Because then I will get to spend more time with—" Then paused, pointed his finger right at my face, and finished, "You."

"North, what are you up to?"

Ben and the lot of us are hanging out in the kitchen right now. Alina's eating dinner; Sean and I are working on the taxes. Just now Ben suddenly turned to North, one of our housemates, and asked, "North, what are you up to?"

Ben is moving fast

Ben is interactive so much of the time now that we really have opportunity to work his social edge and help him grow forward into connection with us. I personally have been doing games built around the idea of school. Each session, I bring in a game that is bookended with my entrance to the room as his second-grade teacher. I start by greeting him: "Hello Second Grade!" To which Ben replies, "Hello, Mrs. Mommy!" which he thinks is hysterical, because at first I was trying to get him to use a fake name, and he totally refused. So now I'm modeling flexibility and humor every day by letting him call me "Mrs. Mommy." Then I sing out, "Benjamin Levin, are you there?" To which he replies, singing, "I am here, Mrs. Mommy!" Then we start our game.

A miracle after a tragedy

Tonight North called from a few towns away to tell us his father passed away today, and that he would be leaving in the morning for Louisiana to make arrangements and show up as needed for his family. I am deeply saddened for his loss and also, selfishly, for our loss—North is an integral part of our family.

Sean and I corralled the children into the activities room to explain what had happened and what it would mean for our family, specifically that we would be losing North for a period of time. Both children were obviously saddened. Ben's questions and comments were remarkable in their compassion and openness:

"Is North sad?"

"Is North disappointed?"

"I'm so sad he will not be here with us."

"Mommy, are you sad?"

"I would be so sad if you two died!"

"I used to think dying was like a man sailing on a boat, but not fishing for any fish. Just sailing on the water. Now I know it's that you go away and you are not yourself anymore."

Then, when North arrived home, Ben walked right up and said to him, "North, I'm very sorry, sorry, sorry, sorry, sorry, sorry that you lost your father." North responded, "I need one of those super-famous Ben hugs!" Ben hugged him for a long time.

WEDNESDAY, MAY 25, 2011

"Don't worry about me!"

Ben got frustrated with me tonight. This week we are visiting a Waldorf school in the town where Sean's office is located. I asked Ben for the umpteenth time if he was feeling okay about visiting a school this week. In response, he exclaimed, "Don't worry about me!" He said it with a certain amount of what—irritation? Desire for independence? Frustration at my relentless talking about what he needs to do to succeed in school? Understandable intolerance of my inability to trust his process and his journey and just get the heck off of his back?

It's a wonderful school, and Ben will visit for three days for us all to see if it is a good fit for him and for the school. Unfortunately, I am not handling it well. I told the teacher today that I was terrified, which was a little inappropriate, because this is about Ben, not me.

And the truth is, Ben is Ben. He is either a fit for the school or not, and he is darn clear that he wants to be there, with other children, and is tremendously eager to be part of a class community. Two years ago Ben was nowhere near ready and seemed, at the time, completely content to be with himself and no one else. Today he is hungry for interaction, and intellectual and social engagement. He wants to be part of a community larger than just the residents of our home.

So when Ben says, "Mommy, don't worry about me!" it just shows he's paying attention and picking up on my insecurities, which are not exactly subtle.

The outcome of the school interviews? It's out of my hands. What will be will be, and at the minimum, it is great to have hope. At the maximum, it is tremendous to be part of Ben and Alina's lives. I know it all will come clear, and wherever Ben ends up, it will be great.

SUNDAY, JUNE 12, 2011

*Changes in Ben**

Some significant changes in Ben over the past few months:

1. *Toileting.* Before IVIG, Ben experienced severe contamination phobias. First, if there were even a drop of urine or a tiny dirt mark (poop or otherwise), Ben would have to have someone else come to clean the area before he could use the toilet. Also, if he were having a bowel movement, Ben needed to flush the toilet every time

---

* In early June 2011, Ben underwent his third IVIG treatment.

he passed even the tiniest of stools. This resulted in flushing up to twenty or even thirty times per bathroom visit. Thirdly, when Ben had a bowel movement, he needed to remove all of his clothing, right down to his socks.

All of these behaviors have completely disappeared for months now. It's like they were never here.

2. *Responsiveness.* Ben's auditory-processing delay is gone. Except, that is, for the typical eight-year-old's "I-don't-feel-like-answering-you" delay. But if Ben chooses not to respond to a question or request, as soon as we up the ante, Ben "miraculously" emerges from his nonresponsive state. For example, I ask, "Ben, are you hungry?" No response. "Okay, Daddy, you can eat Ben's cheeseburgers." Suddenly Ben appears: "I'm here! I'm hungry!"

3. *Interest in others.* Not only is he appropriately responsive to most questions, Ben is also frequently solicitous of others and their well-being. He wants to know how others are feeling, and if they are sad or frustrated, how he might be able to help them feel better. If Alina, for example, wants something to eat and Mommy says no, dinner is over (or whatever), Ben will fly to Alina's defense. "Mommy, you're not being fair to Alina! You're not being nice! Here, Alina, take some of mine!" It's the sweetest thing.

4. *Eye contact.* Ben constantly exhibits firm, continuous, and unsolicited eye contact. He understands now that eye contact is required to get people's attention, and will frequently come over and look me right in the eyes to get my attention. (Note to myself: It's humbling for me to see how often I, myself, don't give eye contact to him or Alina when I'm preoccupied with work, talking on the phone, or just otherwise self consumed!)

5. *Self care.* Ben dresses himself, often choosing his own quite well-matched outfits. He brushes his teeth on his own and does a decent job. He cleans up after his meals and deposits his plates, silverware, and cups in the sink. He is usually willing to clean up his toys, especially if I make a game out of it with the children.

6. *Pill swallowing.* He's a champion, which makes life a heck of a lot easier when it comes to swallowing probiotics, digestive enzymes, and other supplements!

7. *Talking on the phone.* Ben now calls people on the phone (especially Daddy) and talks intelligibly to them. He is able to sustain many conversation loops, even on Skype with his grandparents. His language is more relaxed and less formal, and he uses common expressions such as "that's really cool," or "no problem," and the like. Playdate friends call Ben on the phone, and he has fun conversations with them.

8. *Decreased anxiety.* One of the most stunning changes is the absence of anxiety in Ben. Before his Son-Rise Program and particularly before the IVIG treatments, Ben definitely showed anxiety on a regular basis. Now, Ben goes to school assemblies with tons of loud, screaming, and boisterous children right in his face, as well as parks, playgrounds, beaches, and pediatricians' offices on a regular basis, and is downright gregarious. Moreover he is friendly, but seems to understand others' need for personal space and keeps a reasonable and appropriate distance as he introduces himself, asks them questions about themselves, and interacts with clear enjoyment of the experience.

9. *Literal vs. figurative language.* Slowly but surely, Ben is beginning to understand the difference between literal language and expressions. Before, if I used a figurative expression or hyperbole, Ben would say, "That's not right! You're wrong!" I might say, for example,

"I'm starving to death!" and Ben might respond, "Mommy, don't die! I'll get you some food!" Now, if I exaggerate or use a figure of speech, Ben often asks, "Is that an expression?" with a little grin. One of the hallmarks of autism, and especially of children with Asperger's syndrome, is an inability to understand the subtleties of figurative language and context in communication.

We are definitely making strides—and I mean that figuratively!

WEDNESDAY, JUNE 15, 2011

My son played Scrabble with me yesterday. Real Scrabble. By the rules. With some great words! I have to be one of the happiest mommies in the world. My entire family is obsessed with words, including my parents and my husband. Now my son is playing Scrabble. Ha!

Autism diagnosis, I bite my thumb at you!

THURSDAY, JUNE 16, 2011

Today we had some tough news; the school we had wanted dearly for our BenBen to attend didn't feel the fit would support him or the class. So they said no and encouraged us to apply again next year.

As if that wasn't bad enough, I did a terrible job of telling Ben about the rejection. Ben had Brain Balance today, and I drove him to the appointment. I was in a state of shock and terrified about Ben's reaction. We were almost there when suddenly I blurted out, "Ben, we heard back from the school today, and they told us that you can't go there this fall." There was dead silence. Then after a few moments, "What? They did? Why?" "I don't know, baby," I replied. "I'm so sorry!"

We drove along quietly for another two minutes before we reached Brain Balance. Ben announced, "I'm not going in." "You have to, sweetheart, it's time for your appointment." "I'm not going in," Ben repeated. I was frustrated and beyond furious with myself for giving Ben the news in such a cowardly, impulsive, and thoughtless way. I should have waited, sat on the floor with him, looked him right in the eyes, held his hands, and told him. I wanted to die; I really did. "Ben, I'm sorry," I said. "Let's just do the session, and then we can go home and talk about the school's decision." Ben got out of the car and went inside the clinic. Once inside, he burst into tears: heaving, overwhelming, piteous tears. He lay on the ground and sobbed. The Brain Balance staff looked at me, wonderingly. I tried to calm Ben down, but he was inconsolable. Finally we left and drove home. Ben cried the rest of the day.

Later, I felt really down and shed a few tears. Alina heard me and called out, "Mommy, why are you crying?" I told her, "Because Ben didn't get into school." Alina looked at me, with her enormous blue eyes very serious, and said, "Mommy, you have to remember what you told me. That if Ben didn't get into this school, it's because God knows that he will be so much happier somewhere else!"

Alina had also told me last week she wanted to go to the school even if Ben didn't get to go, and she followed up her comments to me today with, "Mommy, I also will change my mind, if you want me to. I will change my mind and go where you want me to, if you want me to change. Because I know that the best place for me is where my mommy and daddy want me to be!"

How could I stay sad after that?

Tonight I told Alina, "Honey, you really helped me today to feel better." She responded, "I know." I then said, "Yes, but I want to thank you. Thank you so much." Alina paused and then said, "Thank *you*." I asked her, "What are you thanking me for?" Alina replied, "For everything. For everything you do for me."

I don't think my heart can take much more today.

So tonight we are exhausted and angry. We're not angry at a person or a school or anything like that. We're angry that we have to work more, research more, that Sean will have to miss more work, and that the situation is still unclear. We don't frankly know if any school will accept Ben yet, despite his amazing progress and his uncanny beauty of spirit, mind, and heart.

FRIDAY, JUNE 17, 2011

A most meaningful loss

I did think, as Ben was crying today about not getting into the school, "It's okay for him to be unhappy. He's actually caring enough about relationships that he wants them and feels disappointed because he is invested!" Actually, it's even better than that. This loss represents a milestone for Ben. Most kids, by the time they reach Ben's age, have experienced a lot of disappointments. Toughening-up moments. Learning that life's not fair. Getting stronger inside because they discover through each disappointment, each hurt, each loss, that they can keep going, that the thing didn't wreck them, that more good stuff came afterwards, and that they didn't have to be afraid just because life knocked them down for a minute.

Not so for Ben. He has experienced pretty much no disappointments in his life. He has had daily tantrums, frustration when he was neurologically overtaxed and couldn't exert control in an unpredictable and overwhelming world. But that's different. He kind of created that, as a way to exert a sense of control. He was *el presidente* of his self-made world. But this loss was different, not getting into this school. This one was more akin to not getting called up to play on the baseball team or not getting into the school play. This loss came from investment, attachment, and excitement over the opportunity for relationships and participation in a community of children. Any child might have felt the way Ben felt today. It was more like the normal losses and disappointments that most children experience. He rode the wave of his emotions, crying, then angry, and then finding some willingness to accept. He even asked me if there was a camp at the new school we are exploring, because then he could meet some of the kids from that school before school starts in the fall. He walked through the process authentically and with grace.

But that's not actually why I find this so amazing and such a significant moment for him in his recovery. It's that Ben is really in life now, and starting to feel, as we all do, the price of the investment, the ultimate cost of loving, which is to possibly lose or not ever get the thing you want and love. He's connected with others and wants that connection to continue. Despite the bruising.

This loss is Ben's first meaningful loss based on love.

WEDNESDAY, JUNE 22, 2011

Blog from Sean!

"Today, Ben talked to me on the phone. That alone is a great, new development. Then he told me he missed me and loved me. My son is expressing his feelings, his emotions, and where he is in the world. I love that Ben wants to be in our world, and that I am a gateway by which Ben wants to join the world."

MONDAY, JUNE 27, 2011

This afternoon was "Mommy and Alina Day," our weekly time together when I devote myself to Alina. It's an important time each week for both of us, our special time, when Ben is irrelevant and Daddy is also offstage. Today was a very big day: our first visit to the American Girl Doll store, here in Boston. An hour there, an hour back, and two and a half joyful hours in between, complete with a "mini-ice-cream-cone trio," a visit to the salon for Alina's American Girl Doll, and a second mortgage required to pay for said doll's new bed and fancy new dress with matching hat and shoes. It was total heaven, start to finish. Alina was patient, delightful, adorable, and a wonderful buddy. She is my favorite gal pal.

Ben had his third IVIG treatment a few weeks ago. For the past two or three days, Ben has been in a different state than during the past three to four weeks. During the past three to four weeks, Ben was exhausted, chose to connect with us only intermittently, and, for prolonged periods of time, seemed reluctant to exert himself. This all felt normal, as in what we saw after the two other IVIG treatments—incredible fatigue followed within two to four weeks by tremendous behavioral and relational jumps forward. But for the past two to three days, Ben has seemed very autistic. He became jealous, rigid, and emotionally out of control at the bike store on Friday afternoon. He nearly burst into tears Saturday morning over an altercation with Alina. During his Brain Balance sessions, he was nonresponsive and undermotivated, causing his doctor to comment that Ben currently reminds him of when he first met Ben six months ago. Most significantly, Ben has returned to ism-ing fairly often during the day, which we haven't seen in months and months.

Meanwhile, back at the ranch, Sean spent the day with Ben. Until today, he had not seen the degree to which Ben has returned to autistic behaviors. Accordingly, when we returned, Sean was visibly upset. He told me Ben had been extremely nonresponsive. I confirmed that Ben has been that way for several days and that his nonresponsiveness does not seem to be the way it has been for the past many months, that is, like an eight-year-old choosing to avoid interaction in order to yank our chains a little. Instead Ben seems oblivious to us. Sean told me, for example, that he fell asleep on Ben this afternoon for a little while, and Ben didn't seem to notice.

So this feels different than the last two IVIG treatments.

WEDNESDAY, JULY 6, 2011

Choosing celebration over fear

We are still seeing ritualized behaviors we have not seen in over a year. I think Ben was really excited about school, had a grueling three days of IVIG treatments (including a follow-up day of vomiting), got knocked down emotionally by the school rejection, and then went onto intense biomedical treatments—all within a period of weeks. I think he became emotionally and physically overwhelmed. So by doing some autism, he is mediating the amount of feelings he has to process. In other words, through autism, he's being brilliantly self-caring. We can celebrate his autism rather than fear it.

FRIDAY, JULY 8, 2011

Because Ben is so much more interactive and responsive in the presence of other children, I wonder if it was actually just the school rejection in June that threw him into this return to autism. Perhaps he finally felt that he was going to be part of something, a normal kid—and then it was snatched away from him. So now, why bother? Why make the effort to do all of the work of being interactive when he's not guaranteed to get to be in the game in the end anyway? He's particularly resisting interaction with Sean and me, which also makes me wonder if he also might be playing us a little bit.

I didn't feel sorry for Ben today. I did wonder, however, if too many so-called "negative" social experiences, before he's built up a good sense of himself socially, could possibly lead him to choosing to check out more. His ism-ing at the meal table has progressively increased all week, and he continues to be quite nonresponsive.

I want to be wise. I want to live in happiness and faith. I say these positive things, and I am sincere when I say them. But I don't choose faith all the time. I have room to grow. So here is my opportunity to practice, in the form of my very special, so very beautiful Ben and Alina, real trust. Love, guide, and let go, as my Son-Rise Program teachers teach me. Let go and be happy! Watch them growing and experiencing, and not be attached to outcomes. Sustain my faith in them, in myself and my maternal wisdom and intuition, and in God.

MONDAY, JULY 11, 2011

I've decided to homeschool Ben and use a Waldorf curriculum. He might have been fine, all things being equal, if the school had felt they wanted to try it out, but this is also a good option, and I think a more gradual one for Ben. I trust a Higher Wisdom than mine is at work here.

Ben cried again today about getting rejected by the school. I was taken aback by his tears. I didn't realize he was still feeling the disappointment. I tried to reframe the situation for him, by drawing parallels between the homeschool program we are planning and the curriculum at the school he had wanted to attend. Ben asked me, "Will they have everything the same?" I answered, "Yes! Almost everything!" I wrote down all the ways that our homeschool will be the same as "real school." Specifically, both will have main lesson, movement, a specific type of painting, blessings before meals (Ben pointed that one out), recess, handwork, cooking, and a teacher trained in Waldorf, who actually has taken classes through the grades. Ben got very excited when he realized how similar the two "schools" will be. I also reminded him that there may be room for him at the other school next year and that we would be applying again there. "But," I told him, "you need to keep up to their level by working very hard in homeschool, so if they do have space for you next year, you won't be behind." He got very excited.

I think when he was rejected by the school, he lost his motivation. He had the wind knocked out of him and decided to check out for a while.

(My modeling of rage, self-righteous indignation, and self-pity didn't help!) But hope for next year restored some of his motivation. He has the capacity to be happy whether he goes there next year or not, and this time I will do a better job of keeping it realistic that he may not get in there next year and that we don't have a guarantee. But motivation is good!

I went on to explain that the most important thing we have to practice this year is learning how to be part of a class in school. Specifically, not speaking out of turn, following the teacher's instructions, taking turns, not making other children or the teacher wait, and being an active part of the class. He nodded his head and seemed to take it in.

What's in a name?

Ben chose a name for our homeschool program: WiSH (Waldorf School at Home). The implicit subtext was not lost on me.

"Fierce wants," as they say, are huge motivators. Worlds are changed through that kind of motivation. Ben is a force of nature when he chooses to be. But he needs motivation. Ben believes he can get what he wants if he works hard for it. Even if he works hard, he still might not get what he wants. Then guess what? He learns about life and grows more. With another year of Ben's Son-Rise Program along with a year of Waldorf homeschool and other opportunities for socialization, Ben will probably go to a wonderful school next fall—wherever it is.

TUESDAY, JULY 12, 2011

Quite suddenly, and with much joy, Ben seems to be "back." In other words, he seems to have let go of most of the autistic behaviors (*e.g.*, nonresponsiveness, checking out, lack of interest or motivation, lack of energy, etc.). He also seems happier. To me, it looks like Ben's belief that he will in fact be part of a school group (the "WiSH Kids!") seems to have restored his hope that he can indeed be part of a community of kids, and even eventually part of the community of kids he wanted so badly to join.

It also may be that something has completed itself in Ben's brain. Maybe it's the IVIG finally completing its process, or maybe some neurological burst from one of our biomedical therapies. Whatever it is, it's very exciting to see him emerge once again and choose to respond to us. Two days ago I asked him several times to pass me a placemat from the drawer right behind him. He didn't respond at all, didn't even seem to hear me. This morning, at Sean's request, he set both our breakfast settings and gabbed with me throughout the meal.

I love investing in my child.

THURSDAY, AUGUST 11, 2011

I remain too subject to my children's happiness or lack thereof, though with definite progress.

For example, Alina ran in this morning, wearing a new pair of shorts I had bought her and squealed, "Mommy, look! They fit!" My stomach clenched; Alina is truly surprised and ecstatic when clothing fits. She's not fat, but she's short with a protruding stomach, and fitting into age-appropriate clothing is often a problem for her. She's only six, and she is already intensely relieved and happy when things fit. This morning I instantly thought, "Oh God, what is going to happen when she's a teenager and can't fit into anything because she's fat!"

I have a definite choice with her: to allow her to go through her living and learning without me responding codependently or thinking that she has to be unhappy the way I was for so many years, when I was obese and before I found recovery. Moreover, my happiness depends on *my* level of trust and acceptance, not on Alina's moods or choices. I continue to practice giving my children to God.

Ben's school plans for the fall

So now I am trying to pull together our Waldorf-homeschool project. It seemed like such a good idea at the outset, but finding interested families who are willing to commit to two days a week of the program has been really hard.

THURSDAY, AUGUST 11, 2011

Yesterday, Ben and I were in the middle of a storytelling game, and Ben was drawing animals on the table. We were discussing families and puppies (the protagonists of his current stories), and I don't remember the exact context, but suddenly Ben paused. He fixed his gaze on me, looked deeply into my eyes, and asked, "Do you miss your brother?" My brother, Danny, died when we were teenagers, after a failed heart operation. The children know all about him, though we don't talk about Danny very often.

Startled, I answered, "Yes, yes, I do, Ben. Sometimes I feel very sad, because I miss him. Thank you for asking." Ben then responded, "I wish I didn't have an uncle who died before I was born." I replied, "Well, you have Uncle Carl [Sean's brother], and all of your extended family uncles, like Uncle Joshua, Uncle Dave, Uncle Jim, and Uncle Po. But it's not the same as family, I know."

Then, just as abruptly as the conversation had begun, it ended. Ben returned to his puppies, looking down at the table and drawing, with little reference to me. But Ben had chosen to ask me about me.

THURSDAY, AUGUST 11, 2011

Last night, the children and Sean were doing nigh-nighs in Ben's room, and Alina asked Sean why Ben needs to get shots. Once a month, Sean drives Ben to Connecticut to see our DAN! doctor, so that Ben can get a shot of glutathione, an antioxidant produced

103

in the body, which is a critical detox agent for the brain. Ben fears and dreads the shots. Sean answered Alina's question by saying that Ben's body doesn't produce glutathione, but Mommy and Daddy and Alina's bodies do.

Suddenly, Ben began to cry. "I don't want to be different," he sobbed. I listened. At first I thought it was just about taking shots, and I listed off several children in our community of friends who have allergies and have to take shots. But he wasn't persuaded; it wasn't about the shots. He went on, "I want to be like other kids. I want to be with them."

So I shifted gears and explained that everyone has something that makes them feel different. Sean volunteered that he was the only one in the family who couldn't have cheese. I reminded Ben that I'm the only one who can never have bread or treats. Soon after, Alina left the room, and I told Ben that Alina is smaller than all of her peers and she feels terribly different because of that, and even cries about it. We all are different, and feel different, in some way.

Ben responded that it wasn't just being different; it was being different with a boo-boo. So I offered the example of a little boy in the class he visited last spring who has a bone disease and had to wear a cast after one of several surgeries this year. Ben responded to my example by sobbing, "But that's different! He gets to go to school, real school, and gets to be in Mrs. R.'s class!"

So there it was, yet again. Ben is still broken hearted over the Waldorf school rejection, still smarts over being refused the keys to the kingdom. I explained that we would apply again next year and that even the teacher there had encouraged me to try again for fourth grade. Ben was surprised; he told me he was confused, and he hadn't realized the teacher had said we should reapply for Ben to go there next year. But Ben also knows that it's not a sure thing and was not persuaded out of his unhappiness.

Ben then decided to write a letter to Nick, a god-being that Ben has devised, to whom he sends letters whenever he is intensely troubled. The letter read as follows (Ben sometimes puts lines between his words instead of spaces and typically writes in all capitals):

"DEAR NICK | TONIGHT | ALINA | ASKED | WHY | I | NEEDED | DOCTOR | SHOTS | DADDY | ANSWERED | THAT | he | MOMMY | AND | ALINA | HAVE | SOMETHING | I | DON'T | I | BEGIN | TO | FEEL | DIFFERENT | DO | YOU | KNOW | ANY-ONE | WHO | FEELS | LIKE | ME | BEN | IN | MASSACHUSETS"

After he wrote the letter, I read it out loud. Then Ben "read" us Nick's reply, making it up as he went along: "Dear Ben, I know a girl who feels like you do. Her name is [X] and she lives in [Y] and she has to get shots. I will tell her about you so that she doesn't feel different anymore." Then Ben said to me, "Now she knows about me and I know about her and we don't have to feel different anymore!" I asked, "So you felt alone before?" He nodded. So Ben found a way to try to convince himself out of his unhappiness, by creating a fictional girl who felt the way he did. But it wasn't over. He was pensive and on the verge of tears the rest of the evening.

Finally he got tired, got under the covers, and pulled them up under his chin, facing the wall. "Good night, Mommy," he said abruptly. "Ben, are you okay?" I asked, for his face still looked troubled, and his lip was quivering. "Good night, Mommy," he repeated. "No," I said. "I'm not leaving until you tell me how you are. I love you." But I wasn't getting any more out of him. He has so much self-respect and dignity and rarely responds to my emotional inquisitions.

Our conversation ended with the following exchange:

"I'm fine. Good night."

"I love you, Ben."

Very softly, "I love you, too."

Then Sean came over to kiss Ben goodnight. I couldn't quite hear what Sean said, but Ben responded by saying, "I feel so loved."

Truly remarkable in this whole process for Ben tonight was that he didn't check out. He didn't shut us out. He was aware of his feelings and chose to express them to us. And these were hard feelings to face, much less acknowledge. He voiced them and dialogued with us, articulately and responsively. A huge feat for any child, much less one recovering from autism.

He is coming to life. As Sean put it tonight, Ben is like Pinocchio, becoming a real boy, aware of his desire to be part of, to be connected to others and accepted by them. He also feels the pain of self-pity and loneliness. I wondered if I have somehow taught him, inadvertently, that he needs the love and acceptance of others to be happy himself. If so, I can try in the future to model the belief that self-acceptance is the only acceptance I need to be happy.

But Ben has come so far on his journey! What incredible self-awareness and expression of desires! What a beautiful prayer he voiced tonight, through this conversation, of wanting connection and love and to be with other children. I pray that Ben receives the self-acceptance and happiness only he can give to himself and that he also be surrounded by love and joy in his community of peers. I also pray to believe in his journey and in Ben himself.

My precocious little girl

Just a note about another part of my heart, my beloved six-year-old, Alina (who is, by the way, spending tonight in the top bunk of her bunk bed for the first time!). Alina remains a delightful, sweet, loving, and bright little girl. She is caring, feisty, fully engaged in life, endlessly creative, generating joy and invention, and, poignantly, deeply understanding about Ben's special needs.

Alina wanted, for example, to get rid of her training wheels, but Sean and I knew that would cause major explosions with Ben, who just started riding a two-wheeler himself. Accordingly, I had a talk with my little girl and explained that it would be better to wait until Ben is not feeling so competitive and constantly tantruming about things. She looked at me, nodded her head, and replied, "I understand, Mommy. I understand. It's okay." I think she was pretty nervous about taking off the training wheels anyway, but she is very understanding.

She and I have a terrific love affair! I am grateful I am not missing this. It would be easy to do so with Ben so constantly center stage.

TUESDAY, AUGUST 16, 2011

Our Waldorf homeschooling is going quite well. I have set up a hybrid Waldorf homeschool–classroom program, two to three days a week, at our home with a retired Waldorf teacher named Claudine. As of today, we have five to six children who have enrolled, and Ben will have a little "class" to call his own and in which to learn those social skills that he needs to build. We will be starting in September and running for the school year. I am contemplating critical pieces for Ben to work on this year. Clearly, he needs to learn to be part of a group and conform to the social requirements of the classroom. We had several of the children over today, and Ben was so, so happy. It was a delight to see.

SUNDAY, AUGUST 21, 2011

The value of consequences
Tonight Ben didn't want to stop reading for bedtime. Sean and I told him the consequence would be no bedtime stories. Ben chose not to stop anyway and then had a temper tantrum of colossal proportions when we followed through with the consequences and refused to

allow him to have bedtime stories. Sean was magnificent. He grew up in a home with excellent repercussions for defiance and lack of discipline. I had such a violent temper that my parents simply chose to avoid my explosions by caving. I was a good kid, but fundamentally undisciplined and lazy.

I followed Sean's lead tonight, learning as we went. We followed through despite Ben's strong, emotional reaction. I was actually more committed to following through at one point in the evening than Sean was. *I believed that if we gave Ben what he wanted—caved—after Ben cried, we would be sending him the message that all he has to do to get his way is be unhappy. Moreover, we would be teaching him that unhappiness is a way to get what he wants in life.* So although initially I tried to negotiate with kind words (which went nowhere), I soon focused on the need for Ben to learn that his actions have consequences. Sean and I were a good team, and it was a great experience for us as a couple. Ben cried himself to sleep. I was okay, but it wasn't fun.

Flash forward nine hours . . .

This morning, when I came down after my program phone calls and quiet time, Ben was sitting on the couch in our family room. I went over to kiss him good morning, and we had a conversation.

First, Ben said, excitedly, "Mommy, I did something nice!"

"I can't wait to hear all about it, Ben!" I replied. "What did you do?

"Well, Daddy asked me to come somewhere. Can you guess where?"

"Was it breakfast?" I asked.

"Yes!"

"And were you reading?"

"Yes!"

"And what happened?"

"I thought about how last night Daddy asked me to come up-stairs, and I didn't, and I didn't get my bedtime stories, and so today I listened, and came over to breakfast!"

I am so proud of him. He learned. Thank goodness we followed through, or I would never have seen his ability to grow in this way. Both he and Alina continually exceed my expectations, in their goodness, intelligence, and endless capacity to change.

WEDNESDAY, AUGUST 24, 2011

Alina in the playroom: what I used to do

Alina has been in the playroom with Ben and me for most of this week, since camp is over but school has not yet started. Since we started Ben's Son-Rise Program, I have always taken the approach that Alina is second priority in the playroom. It's his therapy room, in a manner of speaking, and Alina does not need therapy. Accordingly, I have always felt that in the playroom I should always give Ben control and let Alina suck it up (for lack of a better term).

Alina in the playroom: a new approach

Tonight, however, I had a video-feedback session with William, my Son-Rise Program teacher, where he advised me otherwise. The crux of William's advice was that Ben is now at a stage where he needs to share the control, share the stage, and be more of a friend—even in the playroom and even to Alina. William advised me that when Alina is in the room, I should use the dynamics that arise to have Ben stretch his social skills. Specifically, Ben doesn't always have to get his way and shouldn't always get to have my attention. Moreover, I can encourage Ben to play with Alina in a flexible way, share things, do things her way sometimes, and share the stage when it comes to getting my attention.

This is really different for me. This is new. For so long I have been afraid to not give Ben all the attention he wants whenever he wants it. I even said to Alina today in the playroom that when we are in Ben's Son-Rise Program playroom, we let Ben be in charge, and he's always in control. I didn't feel comfortable saying that to her, because Ben's not so autistic now and Alina knows it. Now it feels like Ben gets to have more attention and more control just because he's Ben! I could feel the unfairness of my comment as I said it. I even thought to myself in that moment, maybe Alina should have her own playroom? To make it fair.

I'm not saying Ben doesn't still need a playroom or that he's done with autism. But when Alina is there, it's a different scenario now that he has progressed so far. When we are one-on-one with Ben in the playroom, it's still about giving him the space to be totally at ease, without any judgment or direction coming at him, and letting him rest and be in his own world the moment he lets us know he needs to.

But when Alina is there, it's more of a playdate situation, where Ben needs to step up socially and practice the wonderful social skills he's developing. If Ben gets upset, he can get upset. That's okay. Then we just apply certain principles: I can be happy even if Ben is choosing unhappiness at this moment. When he's ready, he'll choose happiness again. I can ask questions, help him to see where he is holding beliefs that lead to feelings of unhappiness. And so forth. But I can stay happy and comfortable even when Ben is not.

I have been so afraid not to give Ben what he wants at all times, because I am afraid of losing him again. The Son-Rise Program taught me that Ben's autism was not my fault, that it was no one's fault, and that it was Ben's way of processing a massive load of stimulation from a world that was neurologically overwhelming to him. I let go of anger at myself for any past parenting misdeeds, and we moved onward into his Son-Rise Program and his recovery. But at times I still pick up the fear that he will reject me again, that he will choose to discontinue our connection, for whatever reason.

Continuing to hold a fear that Ben will stop loving me and wanting to be with me is irrational. Ben loves me deeply and expresses it frequently now, both with hugs and kisses as well as verbal affirmations. He doesn't turn on and off his love for me. He wouldn't return to autism out of anger, either, if I didn't give him his way about something. But my fear that somehow I pushed him into autism remains, only now it's morphed into a fear that I could push him *back* into autism, by failing him in his Son-Rise Program or by failing him as a mother. I still hold on to that fear, to the belief that my best isn't enough, and ultimately to a belief that it's me, not God, who will determine Ben's destiny. Whew, that is a heavy load to carry. No wonder I get tired so much!

On some level, I also know that I am doing the best I can, even if I am filled with an oversized sense of my own power and a healthy dose of perfectionism. With acceptance comes a willingness to change, and I need to let go of these twisted beliefs now, even though the temptation to go back to them might arise now and then. Otherwise, I will hold both of us back. I won't be willing to give him the loving and firm direction and parenting he needs. Moreover, I will hold myself back by thinking that I have to hold on so tightly to Ben and his happiness in order to be happy myself.

MONDAY, AUGUST 29, 2011

Alina has minor surgery tomorrow, to remove some scar tissue. She's a little nervous. Tonight after prayers and singing, Ben came into her room and announced that he wanted to read her a story to "chase away any bad dreams." He read her *Guess How Much I Love You.*

One other note: Ben is again picking up nuances of vernacular. Specifically, he has started to employ the colloquial usage of the word "like" in his sentences, as in, "Alina was saying, like, can we go now?" He uses it with a consciousness of the usage, not the way we all do, *unconsciously* abusing the English language (this is my father speaking now, mind you), but with a self-consciousness that he is using language to be cool, the way cool kids do. Ben wants to be cool. He talks about things and people being cool. Ben has also fallen in love with the expression, "Seriously." Again, he uses it to be cool, sound normal, and be charming. Which it is, coming from him. For example, "You're not doing the right thing, Mom. Seriously." It's adorable.

It's a subtle thing, the use of current vernacular. It signifies that he has paid attention to the language of others and that he is listening to and aware of others.

TUESDAY, SEPTEMBER 13, 2011
Day 1: Ben's first day of homeschool
Today was Ben's first day of his new school, WiSH. We had seven children. Ben had main lesson with his teacher, Ms. Claudine, from 10:30 to 11:30, and was a total rock star. No checking out whatsoever. He did math games, a verse, marching, and painting, and stayed totally present.

Then from twelve o'clock to three o'clock, the other children were here. We had an opening circle and verse outside in the driveway, on this gorgeous and sunny day. Then the children came inside, took off their shoes, and came upstairs to the second floor, where they met Ms. Claudine at the stairwell. One by one, they approached Claudine, shook her hand, and said, "Good afternoon, Miss Claudine!" Then they each climbed the stairs—stairs adorned with glass vases filled with the wildflowers from our garden—into our newly Lazured

WiSH schoolroom. We had an opening verse by the children, which they read, and then a responsive verse by the grownups, which we read to the children as we stood around them in a circle. Next the children went through games, stories, and various activities—including a game with Hendrik, our new au pair from Germany, in which they learned the words for hot, cold, and warm in German. The entire time, Ben stayed with the group.

Tonight he had a meltdown about a book he wanted, which we accidentally recycled a few weeks ago. It lasted about twenty minutes, and he ultimately came up with a resolution: he took magic markers and drew the pages of the book he was searching for and then used those drawings for the game he had wanted to play. I wish I let go of things that swiftly and creatively.

I personally am ready for a case of Valium. I was extremely nervous this morning and felt like I was juggling 5,000 things that "needed" to get done. But Ben had a good day today. It was the beginning of a very special journey for him, back into the world of community with other children.

THURSDAY, SEPTEMBER 15, 2011

Day Two: Ben's first Nature Wednesday

Yesterday was Day Two of Ben's new program. Tuesdays and Thursdays are WiSH School, with five other children at the house. Ten to eleven is main lesson with Miss Claudine and Ben alone (with me observing and facilitating as needed), eleven to twelve is a break for an hour of Son-Rise Program playroom time, and noon to three is WiSH School with the other children for verse, games, painting, handwork, drama, and the other activities Miss Claudine has in store.

Wednesdays are Nature Wednesdays at Miss Claudine's house in Concord. Claudine and her husband live on a pond, and on

Wednesdays Ben, Hendrik, and I journey down to Concord for an-other hour of main lesson, a lunch break, and then a ninety-minute nature experience, which will also include some clay or beeswax modeling. There are three or four other boys who will be part of that. Friday mornings we have eurythmy* and wet-on-wet painting at our house, for one hour, with two of the same children on Wednesday.

Yesterday, as I said, was the second day of this new rhythm, and Ben did well. He got upset when he thought that the other boys were excluding him because they all sat on the same side of the table at snack, with Ben and Miss Claudine and some younger children on the other side. He spent twenty to thirty minutes crying and talking to me about it. He was very open about his assumptions and his feel-ings, and then he told the other children that they were "meanies." He then apologized and asked the mothers to tell the kids that he had felt left out. Then we left, and Ben fell asleep for at least half an hour.

SUNDAY, SEPTEMBER 18, 2011

This morning at 6:15, I asked Ben if he wanted an apple. He said, "If you make it a Honeycrisp, it's a deal!"

From my son who never responded to me.

SATURDAY, SEPTEMBER 24, 2011

Bow Wow Camp!

Ben is traveling, during this new adventure into child society, back and forth between intense responsiveness and total fantasy. He created a fan-tasy world called "Bow Wow Camp," and announced earlier this week that he would be spending the weekend, from Friday to Monday, there.

---

* A movement therapy developed by Rudolf Steiner and used in Waldorf schools.

This weekend each room on our second floor has transformed in his mind into a separate area of Bow Wow Camp. Our third floor, also our WiSH classroom, has become the bedroom for the ten to fourteen puppies that attend BWC, and, accordingly, Ben has slept there for the past two nights. Tomorrow night will be his final night sleeping there. He has eaten most of his meals upstairs at the "camp," and I heard him talking to the "campers" as he went about his business this evening.

He is handling this transition back into intense socialization with other children well. We had only two relatively short meltdowns this week, as opposed to three to four last week. Moreover, they lasted only twenty-plus minutes, which is nothing compared to the daily and lengthy explosions of Ben's past.

Alina wants to be part of WiSH.

Ben wants to be at Alina's Waldorf School.

Of course.

I am happy it is bedtime.

THURSDAY, SEPTEMBER 29, 2011

Two quick sound bites from Alina:

1. Several weeks ago, Ben was bothering Alina, trying to provoke a reaction from her. She responded by saying, "Ben, you know I am the only one who can make myself unhappy!"

2. Yesterday morning, Sean and I were arguing about nothing whatsoever. We sent several escalating comments back and forth, and I suddenly looked at Alina, concerned that we were doing this in front of her. Not missing a beat, Alina exclaimed, "Don't worry, Mom. I'm not learning how to fight!"

She understands so much.

WiSH Week Three

Tomorrow will be the end of our third week of WiSH. Ben is still doing well. One of the WiSH children, however, the only boy Ben's age, has dropped out. I was upset and tried to keep perspective, but I'm scared. It is fascinating to observe Ben as he processes this new onslaught of social stimuli. He is constantly tired. I remember, watching him, that Ben had little to no social contact at all for the past three years, and now he is experiencing a substantial group of children in varying settings—some very unfamiliar—four days a week! Not including the additional playdate scenarios, like the one we had today at a friend's home, with five other children!

Often he becomes nonresponsive but seems still aware of what is going on. One of Ben's challenges is to speak out loud in a clear voice. He often speaks in a very low voice, almost just to himself. It's as though he thinks he's talking out loud, when he's actually not. So we try to help him have an awareness of clear and outward verbal expression.

We are also working on clear handwriting, upper and lower case letters, and punctuation. He is learning handwork, starting with finger knitting. I was surprised and impressed with his patience. He and I spent almost twenty minutes in our main lesson session last Monday figuring out the finger knitting.

SATURDAY, OCTOBER 1, 2011

Ben had a glutathione shot yesterday, and seemed practically neurotypical. I told Sean I want to plant a glutathione tree in our backyard, so we can juice Ben once a week with the stuff. I hope Ben will produce his own glutathione someday, so that he can sustain the wonderful benefits he receives from the shots on his own, without supplementation. Until then, we do the shots.

I've noticed lately that Alina has been compulsively picking at herself. She gets a lot of mosquito bites, and she tends to fall fairly often, leaving little cuts and scratches. She also gets occasional blemishes on her face. All of these areas she picks at until she breaks the skin, leaving little scabs. She has three on her face now, in addition to her recovering wound on her face from some minor surgery a few weeks ago. This morning I put little clear, round Band-Aids on them to help her not to pick at them, but by the end of the day, the Band-Aids were off and so were the scabs. She looks a bit like she is getting over chicken pox.

Truth be told, Sean and I both tend to be a little compulsive that way. So I don't know if the picking is somewhat an outward message that Alina is somehow not comfortable in her own skin, or that she's just the daughter of two compulsive people and she got the gene. I'm not sure how to help her, in either case, other than to pay close attention to her and invest in her by being present when I'm with her and making sure to spend enough time with her.

It is so hard, sometimes, parenting both, because I feel like I give it all to Ben, and then when Alina arrives home at the end of the day, I feel like I have nothing left to give. But I want to be a good mother to both of my children. They both matter.

MONDAY, OCTOBER 3, 2011

I sent out emails to many of the parents from the third-grade class at the school yesterday to invite the children to Son-Rise Program playdates with Ben. Six parents responded! Ben is very interactive and bright-eyed right now. This morning we did main lesson for a full hour. We did finger knitting, writing, verse, stomping, hand clapping, and math problems with beanbags. He worked very hard. I was in heaven.

A penny seems to have dropped again; he is so "with it." I hope it is "sticky" progress and not just temporary effects of the glutathione shot last week. Either way, it's wonderful to experience Ben so present and interested in others. A dear friend, who hasn't seen Ben for almost a year, was over today for a visit and said to me, "He is a different boy! Wow!" Felt great. Ben saw her here, did a double take, and said, "Hi, Auntie Elissa!" while looking right into her eyes.

Earlier this morning, he said to me, "Mommy, I think I know why the school didn't let me in. I think I did some wrong things when I visited there." Internally gaping, I asked him, "Really? What things?" "Well," continued Ben, "I spoke out of turn during main lesson. I think that was wrong. And I think I did some other things that were wrong too."

"Well, Ben," I responded, "You may be right. You definitely need to not talk out of turn during main lesson. There were other issues, but I'm sure you are right. And that is what we can practice this year in WiSH, so you can learn what you need to for when you go back to visit next year!"

Re-energizing our Son-Rise Program

With everything going on with homeschool and WiSH, we have been doing much less time in Ben's Son-Rise Program playroom. But today I posted an ad for a new Son-Rise Program person and got wonderful applicants. I am eager to start digging in deep to Ben's Son-Rise Program again.

Alina has a stomach virus today, but she is in great shape. The marks on her face, about which I was so concerned, are healing, and she is not picking at them. She misses her grandparents very much and is eager to see them. She is such a loving and adorable child.

TUESDAY, OCTOBER 4, 2011

I am so excited. I just bought the whole family tickets to see the Nields, one of our total favorite kids' bands, at Club Passim in a few weeks. We are at this point—going as a family to a concert of children's music. I can't believe it. We can do things like this now.

WEDNESDAY, OCTOBER 12, 2011

I am away at a Son-Rise Program course, and this morning Ben and I talked on the phone:

"Hi, Mommy."

"Hi, BenBen! How are you?"

"Fine."

"I'm so glad, sweetheart. Hey, I miss you a lot, Ben."

"Mommy, I miss you, too."

"Thank you, baby! Have a wonderful day, and I'll talk to you later."

"Bye."

"Bye!"

I miss you, too?

Then tonight, he actually told me about some of his day at school. Tangibles. He lost one of his toys, and his friend, Nigel, helped him find it. Despite Ben's progress, I still harbor a fair amount of negative beliefs:

- I can only be happy if Ben is happy and recovers.
- My life will begin when our Son-Rise Program ends.
- Until that time, I can't take care of my own needs and wants.

No wonder I constantly feel exhausted, irritable, and victimized. *I am my own victimizer.* I am trying to replace these beliefs with the idea that I can actually only help Ben if I put my own well-being first, and that regardless of Ben's happiness, I can be well and peaceful within. Working on it.

An email from Ben's WiSH teacher, Miss Claudine, about class today:

Hello Susan,

We have a new goal. Ben needs to respond to me if I ask him a question. I told him it can be "I don't know, wait a minute while I think," but at least some recognition I was talking to him. I was thinking perhaps he can put his hand to his head to let me know he is thinking about the answer, and he will come up with something.

Lots of eye contact this week. So nice.

Love,

Claudine

WEDNESDAY, OCTOBER 19, 2011

Samuel

On Monday, we hosted Samuel for a playdate after school. It is very complicated with Alina, and I have to get clear about my purpose, because she feels very left out and dismissed by me. In any case, Samuel and Ben did a scavenger hunt in the playroom, with me facilitating. It was a blast. It went on too long, but the boys worked really hard—the clues involved things like jumping jacks and crab walking together and lots of fun challenges. Each of the clues got them to find a cardboard bone with the name of one of the class's children on it. Once they found all the bones, they were done. There were fourteen bones! Samuel was pooped, but I think both boys had a great time.

As they were leaving, all I could think was, "Will they come again? Was this too weird? Do we seem desperate? Does Ben seem autistic?"

Jennifer

Then today we had a playdate with Jennifer (not her real name), a sweet nine-year-old girl. The first hour went well. I did a scavenger hunt with Ben and Jennifer while the younger children (there were four of them, including Alina) spent time in the WiSH classroom with Hendrik. The scavenger hunt was awesome. On beautiful paper, I wrote out eight challenges that Ben and Jennifer had to complete together in order to earn their clue to where the prizes (SCD [Specific Carbohydrate Diet] almond-flour-and-honey cookies wrapped in foil) were located. These were some of the challenges:

- Ben and Jennifer had to make sounds and movements like an animal for the other to guess;
- Ben and Jennifer had to pretend to be characters from the Garden of Eden and act out some version of the story (the third-grade Waldorf curriculum includes Old Testament stories, including the Garden of Eden);
- Ben and Jennifer had to create a story about fairies; and,
- Ben and Jennifer had to draw a picture of their fairy story and then retell the story to us using their drawing as a visual aid.

And so on. They worked beautifully together. Ben was responsive, engaged, and clearly enjoyed spending time with his new friend.

After the scavenger hunt, I made the mistake of inviting Ben to show Jennifer the WiSH classroom. At that point, Alina took over somewhat, and Ben got upset about the little kids invading his time with Jennifer. He asked me repeatedly, "Can we have alone time again, Mommy?" I tried explaining that sharing time with friends, even friends we don't want to be with, is part of learning to be in school and having community with other kids, but he was pretty miffed. But he went with it, had no tantrum, no meltdown, no sad tears, none of that. He just did his best. He was awkward. He pushed too hard and asked them all to play games that made no sense given the context of the group, and the younger children clearly thought he was from Mars. Then the group came downstairs, where Ben was even *more* awkward.

How do I feel about my awkward kid?
I don't give a hoot! I am so proud of my son right now. A day like today: total exhaustion, an unexpected convergence of small children,

and more social stimulation than he's probably had in his lifetime—and he stayed with it. Stayed responsive. Stayed open. Listened to my suggestions and guidance. Shared Jennifer. Let go.

Ben loves this class of children at the Waldorf school. More than that, he loves connecting with other people. He loves connecting with me, his daddy, and his sister. As for the social skills, I'd be awkward too if I had spent no time with other children for a very long time. I want to enjoy every moment—even the nervousness, the anxiety, and the butterflies in my stomach when the playdate is over and I don't know how the other family feels about us. There's plenty of time to learn.

I don't know if Ben will be accepted at Waldorf next year. I can't think about that right now. Fear's target is always in the future, and I have no interest in focusing on fear. What's happening right now is hopeful and exciting. We are finally in the game. This is what we've worked for.

THURSDAY, OCTOBER 20, 2011

Tonight Alina, Ben, and I were awaiting Sean's return from a business trip. I was reading the children a story in our bed, and the three of us were cuddling. Ben lay by my side, snuggling up to me and stroking my hair. Alina lay on my other side, also cozy and snuggly. I felt like I were in some afterschool-special movie about families! On top of that, Ben is actually asleep right now in our bed. Never before has Ben chosen to stay in our bed and fall asleep there.

I think it is the recent increase in the mitochondrial supports—ubiquinol, specifically. Also, Ben has decided that Waldorf is, to use his words tonight, his "favorite school on earth." Our WiSH teacher expressed her concern to me this afternoon that he is too fixated on getting into the school next fall. Sean and I share her concern.

As a motivating force, however, Ben is driven by his intention to get in next year and is consequently working hard on his responsiveness, eye contact, cooperativeness, and overall willingness to interact. So for now, I'm not going to quash his excitement, though I did talk to him tonight about the possibility that the school might reject him again next year. I also told him that in my opinion, he can be happy regardless of what school he attends. I asked him if he thought he could be happy regardless of whether he goes to his "favorite school on earth." He replied, "A little." He looked very sad at the prospect. But I am going to keep throwing it out there, every now and then, just to keep us all aware that happiness does not depend on anything outside of ourselves.

Ben is much younger socially than other children his age, because of his lack of experience and because the autism retarded his social and emotional development. But he is catching up. Who knows where he will be in April?

SATURDAY, OCTOBER 22, 2011

All this week, Ben had days filled with varying amounts of intense social activities, and we saw little to no ism-ing in response. He's tired, but he is building his social muscles, and his endurance and stamina need time. That's what this year is for.

SATURDAY, OCTOBER 29, 2011

Sweet moments

1. This morning Ben ran into our bedroom and yelled out, "Mommy, I'm so excited!" I didn't even care what words came next. My son was excited about something, and he wanted to tell me about it! I asked, "What, Ben, what are you excited about?" He went on to tell me about a party he had made up, a pretend party with so-and-so characters attending.

2. A few weeks ago, I explained the difference between fantasy and reality to Ben. Sometimes he gets so deeply involved in his

imaginary stories and creations that he appears not to know that the stories are actually fantasy, so I wanted to make sure he knew the distinction. He totally got it, and now he will say, in the middle of an imaginary play he is creating, "But it's only fantasy, Mommy." I also explained that fantasy is not for classroom time (unless the teacher expressly requests an imaginary project for the class), but rather for recess or playtime. Otherwise, Ben needs to focus on the topic at hand in order to be successful in the class, for him to learn the material being presented, and for the teacher to see he is present and really listening to what she is trying to teach him.

3. The other day, Ben had a playdate with a little girl named Auden. I gave them a challenge during a scavenger hunt to come up with a fairy tale together. I left the room to watch through the one-way window in the door and observed them working together. They got distracted at one point by a bunch of cards that were lying around and spent a few minutes looking at them. Actually they were cardboard bones that another person had created for Ben for a theme last year. So they were looking at these bones, when all of a sudden Ben said, "Oops, we're not on task. Let's get back to the fairy tale." I nearly fell over: Ben chose to redirect *himself*!

Ben also came up with a great image during that playdate. At another challenge, I had them telling a story together, tag teaming. For example, Auden would say one piece of the story, then tell Ben it was his turn when she was ready for him to go. Then Ben would tell part of the story, until he wanted Auden to take over. They went back and forth upwards of twenty-five to thirty times. At one point in the story, Ben came up with the image of a boy cursed by a witch so that he had the body of a tree but the head of a boy. Later in the game, I challenged them to draw a scene from their story, and Ben's part of the drawing including the tree boy. I hope he will write books someday.

I am too tired to continue, and there will be many more entries in which I can detail more of Ben's milestones and the ongoing miracle of his interactivity. We still have speech issues (he can't say "th" to save his life, "thank you" comes out as "fank you" and "they" comes out as "day"), energy issues (which we are attacking with ongoing mitochondrial-support work), social awkwardness (don't get me started), and picky, picky, picky eating (getting better). But this is a work in progress; we are not done with our Son-Rise Program, and there is no gun pointed at our head demanding a speedy finish. Perhaps we are in our home stretch, and we have maybe another year, another year and a half. But I'm not looking at the ending. Like my son, I'm enjoying the story.

MONDAY, OCTOBER 31, 2011

A Happy Halloween

Tonight we had a pretty big, intense, emotional time after Ben wouldn't listen to Sean, and Sean's consequence for Ben was that Ben didn't get stories, but Alina did. It was also an intense evening because it's Halloween, and Ben didn't want to go trick or treating because he can't eat any of the candy, and he knows it.

After Sean imposed the consequence of not reading to Ben, Ben cried a lot and then lay in our bed. When I came in to find out what was going on, he told me he thought I loved Alina more than I loved him. Sean said he had no idea how Ben had gone from no stories to Mommy doesn't love him.

I joined him on our bed, where he lay crying a little, and told him that before Alina was born, he took over my whole heart, and when Alina was born, I asked God to make my heart bigger so that I wouldn't have to take any of my heart away from Ben. I told him God did make my heart bigger, so no love was taken from Ben, and I could love Alina, too.

Ben then responded, "I need to make a time machine to go back to when I had your whole heart!" Or something to that effect. "Can I make a time machine? I need to make a time machine!" It was super cute, and I didn't know what else to say, so I just lay there with him. He calls our bed, when he goes underneath our quilt, his "cave." Ben and I lay there in his "cave." I told him there wasn't much air in the cave. I held him and stroked his hair. Then he suddenly said, "I'm so totally happy now, happier than I've ever been before." I blinked, not knowing what he meant or how to respond. I said, "I'm so glad, Ben!" Then he said, "I feel totally loved right now, more than ever." Then he got up out of the bed, closed his eyes, and said, "I'm sleep-walking now back to my room!" And off he went.

I followed him back to his bedroom, where he got into bed. I said our nightly prayers and kissed him. Sean had come in, and Ben told him he (Sean) loved Alina more than Ben, and he knew that because Sean had read stories to Alina tonight and not Ben. Sean responded, "That's not true, but if you want to believe it, you can," and kissed Ben good night.

One more thing. As I said good night to Ben tonight, he replied, "Good night. And happy Halloween!" Happy indeed.

WEDNESDAY, NOVEMBER 2, 2011

Tomorrow is Ben's ninth birthday. We are having a party, because Ben wanted one. Almost all of the children he hoped to be there are coming, upwards of nine to ten kids. We are doing a great, big scavenger hunt, which I will no doubt write about some other night.

The thing I want to share tonight, however, is that tonight when I said good night to Ben, I told him, "Do you know how proud Daddy and I are of you? How wonderful a person you are, and how far you've come? How kind, and loving, and special you are? We are so proud of you." He wrinkled his nose, put his head almost underneath his covers, and said, "When you said those things, you made my day."

He makes mine every day now. I'm not sure autistic is the right word for Ben anymore. He is of course still intensely impaired, but he is no longer living unto himself.

His favorite expression these days is, "Get real!"

What is *real* is that our son is with us.

Happy birthday, BenBen!

THURSDAY, NOVEMBER 3, 2011

A truly great birthday

Well, the party was as good as anyone could have wished for. The whole day can be summed up in Ben's comment to me this evening as I was tucking him in. At the end of prayers when we were thanking God for all of our blessings, Ben spontaneously said, "Thank you. This was the best party I ever had!"

FRIDAY, NOVEMBER 4, 2011

Susan and Sean,

He did so well! I need to tell you and Sean two pieces you missed. When everyone was showing up, I overheard Ben introducing everyone to each other. It was such a sweet gesture and something I would never expect a child to think of or follow through with.

Later, I noticed Nigel was sort of hanging back. I whispered to Ben to keep in mind he didn't know anyone. Ben walked up beside Nigel and continued playing. Later I was on the landing upstairs looking out of the window. I watched Ben as he repeatedly looked over towards Nigel and finally went to stand next to him again. He was so happy everyone was there to play with yet he did not overlook his friend's feelings. What an incredibly sweet child you have! Bravo!

Claudine [Ben's WiSH Teacher]

THURSDAY, NOVEMBER 10, 2011

Trouble in paradise

For the past week, Ben has been in a bit of a mode. In other words, all the social excitement of last week with the birthday party was very stimulating for him, and it appears that he is taking some time to neurologically catch up.

To do this, he has been less connected to others and more engaged in rigid and repetitive behaviors, focusing mainly on imaginary school classes he has created and whose "students" he has developed into meaningful characters. For example, there is one guy named "Joseph," who wasn't allowed to go to the school he wanted to attend even though his sister was. (Subtle.) Then there is a child named "Zack," who likes to be mean to any children younger than second grade. Ben's stories have been largely noninteractive this week, though he has clearly wanted (and demanded) an audience for them.

MONDAY, NOVEMBER 14, 2011

Ben is a little ism-y right now; we had the Martinmas festival/lantern walk Friday evening, and it was a lot of stimulation. Tons of children in a small room together, lots of food Ben couldn't eat, a long walk that started very late in the evening. The whole thing was a lot for the little guy, and he's been somewhat nonresponsive since. He's great in the playroom, extremely responsive and interactive, so it's clearly not a neurological issue, but rather an attitudinal issue. This means that in order to leverage our time with him right now, it's about going at his pace and being really loving and patient, encouraging but not pushy. He will instantly pick up on a caregiver's energy or frustration and go internal. So my approach right now is to be mega-loving, mega-fun, mega-cheerful, and mega-nonjudgmental. Anything he gives, I celebrate.

SUNDAY, DECEMBER 18, 2011

We are in the process of assessing the best educational environment for Ben for next school year, beginning Fall 2012, when Ben will be in fourth grade. We will apply again to the local Waldorf school, where Alina is enrolled and see what happens. Ben's progress through our WiSH program is impressive, and the relationships he has established with peers and his teacher, Claudine, have clearly improved his ability to develop critical social and classroom skills.

Ben wants desperately to attend the Waldorf school. He expects to visit the class again this winter as part of the admissions process, and he's terrified. He has told me and others (including a friend from WiSH, who is Ben's age) how nervous he is and how worried he is they won't "let him in again." I told him that he doesn't have to go, we don't have to apply, and I would even allow him a little television if he chose to continue with WiSH instead of applying (oops). But even with the TV offer—though that did prick up his ears!—he was firm: "No, I really want to go to the Waldorf school. I just love that class."

So our decision is that Ben should have his chance to go for his dream, and if he falls on his bum, it's a great learning experience. He loves WiSH, so there will be a cushion for that bum if they reject him again.

For my part, I'm not sure what the best environment is for him at this stage. On the one hand, there is not as much support in that particular school environment compared to what he gets attending school in his own home. On the other hand, I think Ben's progress would skyrocket if he were given the opportunity to show up for a structured routine and be part of a consistent classroom community. Happiness works, and I think Ben's happiness being there would motivate him to work incredibly hard.

His physical stamina is still lacking, so we continue to work on mitochondrial supports, whole-food supplements, and craniosacral therapy.

Then there is Stoneridge Montessori, located about five minutes from our home, but I don't think their child-driven method would effectively support a child recovering from autism. My intuition tells me to try again at the Waldorf school, and if they say no again, do another year of WiSH and apply again next year for fifth grade.

Alina is another story. She feels a bit lonely, I think, in her small Waldorf classroom with few girls and a bunch of very tightly connected boys. I'm not sure Montessori would be a bad choice for her socially, though I believe the Waldorf curriculum is much better for her in other, more important ways. It is a challenge to parent two children with such profound, important, and *different* needs!

My constant parenting errors

I was impatient and intolerant with Ben this afternoon. We went to the library today. The children always bring home dozens of books when we go, and today was no different. They also always go into another world when we bring home library books and become little reading zombies. Ben in particular was nonresponsive to almost every request I made, because he just wanted to read his new books. Very understandable, but I was feeling tense, and I judged him.

For example, I said to him, "If you don't answer me when I ask you something, I will never take you to the library again!" I said, "You are going to lose your friends if you don't answer their questions when you are reading!" To that comment, Ben replied, with tears, "I am so upset now!" When I said I was sorry for saying that, he said, "Thank goodness; I thought you were saying you wouldn't be my friend anymore." I felt bad about myself, but I didn't stop. I told him, "I'm sorry, it's just when you don't answer me it reminds me of when you used to be autistic and never answered me, and I panic inside a little." Like he needs to hear that. Maybe it wasn't terrible to say that, to at least explain why I was saying such irrational things when he just wanted to read his darn book. I should have taken myself away for a bit till I got my head screwed back on, rather than giving him all that analysis and criticism. Live and learn.

"She needs to learn life isn't fair"

Tonight Sean is traveling, and he will be traveling on business for the next four days. Alina wanted to sleep with me in our bedroom, but I said no, because she snores and I wouldn't get any sleep. Ben, however, wanted to sleep in our bed, and I said it was fine. (He doesn't snore, and, when he does, it's not a foghorn like Alina!)

After Ben left the room, and Alina found out Ben was sleeping with me, she burst into tears and said, "I know it's not right, but I feel sometimes like you do love Ben better than me!" We've had this conversation before. I explained, calmly, "No sweetheart, it's just that you snore and Ben doesn't." She replied, "I know, and I want you to get a good night's sleep, but I want to sleep with you at the same time!" So I offered to not let Ben sleep with me, and she was happy again.

Then I went to kiss Ben good night, and I told him he had to go back into his bed and leave our bedroom. I asked him if he was upset, and he said no. Then he got into his bed, and looked unhappy. He said, "I'm so upset right now!" I felt terrible.

I asked him what had bothered him, and he said to me, "You upset me with three things. First, the things you said to me about not answering and not paying attention. Second, what you said about not being my friend. The third one I won't tell you." I replied, "You have to." So he said, "Just because Alina was jealous, you shouldn't have told me to leave your bed. She needs to learn that life isn't fair."

I was so angry with myself when I heard that. Ben was absolutely right, and I allowed Alina to manipulate me with her unhappiness. *Again.* Ben frowned sadly and wouldn't look at me.

I know he will forgive me, and there is always hope that Alina will grow into choosing happiness despite my (and others') constant reinforcement that unhappiness will get her what she wants. I want to learn from tonight to stay out of the driver's seat, to let my children grow and not try to rescue them. I need to surrender these unfair expectations of them, especially of Ben, that he should "snap to" like some military robot, rather than responding in the best way he can as a nine-year-old boy. Forget the "recovering from autism" part; the kid's just a nine-year-old who wants to not respond sometimes.

My "problems" this evening, however, are all accompanied by underlying miracles. Notably, our current consideration of various options for Ben's schooling contains an unspoken assumption: *Ben is able to be in a school now!* Three years ago, he was nonresponsive, noninteractive, and entirely uninterested in other people. Now he is eager to be part of a classroom community and, most meaningfully, actually has the capacity, in the view of experts, to succeed in a classroom environment.

Also, Ben's communication to me this evening was a miracle. He told me he was upset. He told me why he was upset. He then spoke wisdom to me, namely that life isn't fair, and he applied it in a perceptive and insightful manner to the situation with his sister.

These are all miracles of progress and a reflection of a beautiful soul who has emerged, of his own volition, into human society.

MONDAY, DECEMBER 19, 2011

This morning I went into Ben's room when I saw his light was on and asked him, "How do you feel?" (I was going to ask him, "Are you still upset?" and realized that was inviting a focus on unhappiness. I was glad I realized it before I said it!) Ben waited several moments before answering, during which I did not interrupt him but waited patiently, believing he was taking the time he needed to process the question and his response. (This was a win for Mommy.)

Then he replied, "I have tears in my eyes, so I don't think I feel happy."

I again waited, praying for the right words. Then I asked, "You know you can decide to be happy even if you have leftover tears in your eyes, right?"

He answered, "Yes."

I added, "And you know you can be unhappy and that's fine too, right?"

"Yes."

"Well," I continued, "I've decided to be happy all day today. No more grouchy Mommy!"

"Yeah, like you were yesterday!" Ben said, smiling.

"Yes. Today I am going to be happy, because I get to be with the people I love, you and Alina. And you have a playdate today with Elowyn!" Elowyn is a friend from the school where Ben wants to go.

"Yes! And I have an imaginary sleepover with Cleo, my friend from PBS Kids School!"

"Yes! That is so exciting!!"

By now Ben was grinning ear to ear. I told him, "Ben, I am going to go take quiet time now. Would you like one of your new library books? There's one in our room."

"Yes! I hope it's a Ricky Ricotta!"

MONDAY, DECEMBER 19, 2011

Ben had a playdate today with a girl from the school he wants to go to. Her little sister, who is Alina's age, was supposed to come. The little sister did not, in fact, come. Alina stole the play date; in other words, the older sister who was supposed to play with Ben played with Alina instead. They tried to include Ben much of the time, but he "got it" that the girls had bonded and let them have their girl time together. I asked him how he was doing, and he said he was fine with it and seemed actually not too upset. Until later.

After dinner, Alina, Ben, and I were hanging out at the dinner table. (Sean was away on business.) Suddenly Ben decided to make himself unhappy. He was supposed to have an imaginary sleepover playdate with a girl named "Cleo" from one of his imaginary classes, and "Cleo" was coming over this evening. But Ben suddenly decided that Cleo had to come over on Thursday, the day of the WiSH Hanukkah Festival, which was a total conflict. He started whining, crying, and being unhappy.

I tried to ask him questions, such as, "Why are you deciding to make yourself unhappy? Cleo is imaginary, and you can have her come any night. Why are you deciding to have her come the one night it doesn't work?"

He just kept crying and whining. So I told him it was fine with me if he wanted to be unhappy for a while, although I didn't understand that choice, and I was going to go clean up. Alina took my cue and stayed calm and relaxed, while Ben raged and cried.

A little later Alina went to go poop (an easily fifteen- to twenty-minute window for me to talk to Ben privately). I went into the family room, where Ben was sitting, and asked him to come talk to me. He was still visibly upset. I began asking him questions again, and he continued in the same vein. I asked him if he remembered that Cleo was imaginary. He said yes. I asked him if he remembered the difference between real and imaginary. He said yes, of course, he always knows these children are not real. I asked him why he wants to choose unhappiness right now. He chose not to answer that question, but went back into his rage that the Hanukkah Festival was on the wrong night, and we had to change the day.

I stayed very calm, mostly, and relaxed and comfortable while he was experiencing the tantrum. Then suddenly, Ben said, "It's something else, too. I don't want Alina to have no one here when I have playdates. She steals them."

Aha!

It all became clear. Ben was disappointed in the playdate and used the Cleo/Hanukkah Festival conflict as an excuse to process uncomfortable feelings. (Pretty impressive if you ask me, as most grown-ups would do that with a few martinis or a box of oreos!) Because I didn't judge or try to direct his feelings about any of it, he was eventually able to uncover the underlying reason for his unhappiness. It took a bit of time (and thank God for Alina's healthy digestive system, lol), but he chose to share his pain with me.

I told him if I had a playdate that I was excited about, and my little sister stole it away from me, I would be very disappointed. I asked him if he was disappointed about the girl today, and he nodded. I told him for any future playdates, I would have Alina absent or engaged with some other child. He was pleased and nodded his head vigorously. He seemed much more comfortable and spent the rest of the evening laughing and playing with Alina and me.

I'm starting to get it.

SUNDAY, JANUARY 1, 2012

Ben loves waking up very early, and lately we have had a bunch of 3:30 AM talks and snuggles. I wouldn't miss it for the world.

This morning, however, he "slept in" till 5:00 AM, at which point he woke me up by whispering, right into my ear, "I have something to tell you!" I asked, "What?" with a groggy smile. "Happy New Year, Mommy!"

What a way to start 2012.

WEDNESDAY, JANUARY 4, 2012

Tonight Ben came up to me in the kitchen and told me, "Mommy, I'm sorry we weren't able to play your game today!" I had brought a theme in about Saturn, but he wanted to go outside and have "recess" instead, which was also a lot of fun.

I was touched that he remembered, even hours later, that we didn't get to my game, that he considered my feelings, and chose to come all the way into the kitchen to express love and concern for me, directly to me.

FRIDAY, JANUARY 6, 2012

It is so amazing how much Ben now wants to be with me. It's the most wonderful feeling.

His room has been extremely cold, so he has been sleeping with me in our bed. We had the heat fixed today, so Ben can go back to sleeping in his own room. So tonight, he was unbelievably affectionate. He asked me to hug him "for a whole minute." I did, and then he kissed me on my face about five times, before retiring to his own bedroom. I was touched. He really wanted to stay sleeping in our bedroom, with me. (I know, most people would think, "Duh, what nine-year-old boy doesn't want to sleep with his mom?" Autistic boys, that's who!)

The fact that he wants to be with me, instead of in his own space, his own, alone space—I don't think I'll ever fully get over it. My son wants to be with me and with us.

SUNDAY, JANUARY 8, 2012

Three days ago, we sent in Ben's application for admission to the Waldorf school for this fall. We all had high hopes, based on their emphatic invitation last year to reapply this year and especially given the great strides Ben has made this year in WiSH.

But yesterday we received a letter from the school, notifying us that having received Ben's application on Tuesday, they would be neither admitting Ben, considering his application, nor open to application from him in the future. I was speechless. I showed the letter to Sean, who was furious. We talked abut how to give Ben the news. I wanted to do better this time.

This morning we sat the children down for a family meeting.

Me: Ben, we got a letter from the school yesterday. They said you can't go there.

Ben: Ever?

Me: [pause] Yes.

Ben: [pause] Why?

Me: Ben, I honestly don't know. They didn't give any reason.

Ben: Do you think they're evil?

Sean and I grinned at each other.

Me: [after another pause] Well, honey, we do, a little bit. Yep, we sure do. But really they just don't know how to do this very well.

Ben: [beginning to cry] Then I won't be able to go there?

Me: That's right, baby. And we are going to have a great time in WiSH. But I know this is hard. We will still get to see your friends from the school, if you want to. Do you want to?

Ben: Yes. [continuing to cry]

That was pretty much it. Ben cried for a little while and then seemed to let it go. Sean and I stayed calm. I actually felt relieved. I thought to myself, we don't have to worry anymore. The pressure I have been putting on myself and on Ben is over. I can come back to a Son-Rise Program attitude and stop having an agenda about creating Ben's happiness.

Later we had an interesting conversation at the dinner table. Ben announced, first, that he was going to write a letter to the Waldorf school admissions director, pretending to be the school administrator, telling the admissions director she's fired. Sean and I thought that was great.

Then, Ben announced that under no circumstances would he allow Alina to go to WiSH. He said WiSH was his, and Alina already had a real school, and that it was not fair for her to have both. "She has to go to the school!" Ben stated adamantly.

I asked him, "But Ben, how are you going to feel when Alina is spending time with people in Mrs. Z's class, when you can't ever go to the school yourself?" He replied, "It's really fine. I just don't want Alina to go to WiSH. That's my rule!"

When I told Alina she would be staying at the school, she looked very sad and said, "But Mommy, I want to be with Ben!" I answered, "But honey, Ben wants WiSH for himself." Alina paused and, looking very serious, old, and wise, responded, "Okay."

I saw the comprehension in her eyes and was impressed, as I so often am by my daughter's understanding. She understood Ben's feelings, didn't take it personally, and let go of her desire to be in school with Ben in favor of his desire for her to be elsewhere. She loves her big brother *a lot.*

MONDAY, JANUARY 9, 2012

Ben had more hard feelings today, and now wants to make all the teachers evil so the children will all abandon the school (love it).

Ben also told me he wants to be at a "real" school, and that he will wait for Miss Claudine (our WiSH teacher) to tell him when he has all of the abilities he needs to attend a real school. He cried as he told me this. I assured him we would explore lots of schools and find one that is right for him.

I'm happy he is alive and wanting to be part of a school. I look forward to the day when all of Ben's wishes are fulfilled.

Ben's not the only one who's riding the waves.

TUESDAY, JANUARY 10, 2012

Last night Ben asked me, "What did I do wrong, Mommy? I'm sure I must have done something wrong to make them not take me? What could it have been?" And then later, "Can you ask one of the teachers from the school to come to WiSH, Mommy? Then I can prove to them that I don't interrupt anymore and that I know how to pay attention! Maybe then they might let me come to the school!"

After hearing these questions, I was tempted to choose unhappiness. "My poor son, my poor Ben, the most lovely, brilliant, kind, and friendly child in the world, and those people won't even consider his application!" I was tempted to let his words trigger beliefs about the wrongness of the universe, about how fearful people can damage my son's sense of self, that maybe I should push the school to give him a chance, or at least a visit . . .

But I didn't give in to those thoughts and feelings. I decided to believe that Ben is strong, resilient, and ultimately someone who will choose happiness in his life, and that this experience will strengthen rather than harm him. I also believe it will strengthen me and not harm me, if I choose to believe that this is all part of God's plan.

Moment by moment, I am walking the line.

THURSDAY, JANUARY 12, 2012

I talked to Ben about autism

Today in the playroom, Ben was remarkably affectionate. He wanted nothing other than for me to hug him, tightly, for long periods of time. He also was very willing to play the Spanish fruits and numbers theme I brought in. That was our first session.

During our second session, he was again very affectionate and made amazing eye contact. I wanted to ask him how he was feeling about the process with the school, but bit my tongue because it was a head thing and not an in-the-experience thing. So I held off, and we played. I felt connected to him; he was available, present, and flexible, and he wanted to be with me.

A few minutes later, I decided to invite Ben into a conversation I had never attempted before, namely, about autism, his Son-Rise Program, and my beliefs about his process. He seemed to take it all in.

Me: Ben, would you like to know what I believe about the school's decision?

Ben: [immediately looking directly into my eyes, as he always does the moment I mention anything related to the school] Yes.

Me: Okay. Well now you know you had autism?

Ben: [firmly] Yes.

Me: Do you know what autism means?

Ben: What?

Me: No, I'm asking you, do you know what it means, autism?

Ben: No.

Me: Would you like to know what it means?

Ben: Yes.

Me: Well, in people with autism, their brains work differently than other people. Specifically, they get overwhelmed by talking to people, looking at people, or connecting with people. So they just choose not to do those things. So it's really hard to have relationships, to have friends, and to do certain things. Like, when you had autism, you didn't look at me or Daddy, and you didn't hug us much.

Ben: Oh. I think that's why we did homeschool.

Me: That's right. We do a Son-Rise Program, which we call homeschool, in order to help you learn how to do things you couldn't do when you had autism. So you know how Daddy and I are always saying to you, "Great job looking, Ben! Great eye contact!" and stuff like that?

Ben: [grinning] Yes!

Me: That's because we are so happy that you are learning to look at us, because that's very hard for someone with autism. Eye contact is one of those abilities that you need to develop in order to go to school.

Ben: Oh!

(Ben said to me three days ago that when he had enough "abilities," he would be able to go to school.)

Me: So here's what I think happened at the school. Last year, when we applied there and you went for your visit, you still had some autism, and the school saw that and thought they would not be able to teach you well enough because they don't know how to teach to children with autism. Then this year, when we applied, they decided you probably still had autism, and so they still couldn't teach you. Only it wasn't fair because they didn't give you a chance.

Ben: And they canceled the visit.

Me: Exactly. So look, the school sent us an email saying they knew we were upset and that they would like to meet with us to talk about the letter. So Daddy sent an email back saying we were indeed upset and would appreciate an opportunity to meet and get an explanation for why they rejected us out of hand. So we are going to go and meet with them sometime in the next two weeks and see what the deal is.

Ben: I think it will be difficult to change their minds.

Me: We're not going to try to change their minds. I just want to understand. I also want to know if, when you have no more autism and can do everything children without autism can do, can we apply again?

Ben: Right!

Me: Right. So that's where we are.

At the end of our conversation, Ben gave me a *big* hug.

I am concerned about the nine-year change. I want Ben's sense of himself to remain strong and confident. In Waldorf child-development theory, the year between ages nine and ten is crucial to the child's future development, due to the sense of individuality that emerges at that time. So I am here, 100 percent, to reinforce the beauty, brilliance, and enough-ness in Ben, regardless of this emotional and psychological sucker punch from the Waldorf school.

TUESDAY, FEBRUARY 7, 2012

Sean and I were in bed with the kids at nigh-nighs, and Alina had fallen asleep, snoring away peacefully. Sean and I were discussing Alina's weight, and that we weren't sure if she had lost any weight on her new GAPS (Gut and Psychology Syndrome) regimen, but that she seemed healthier and not as obsessed with food after being on the plan for a few weeks now.

Ben suddenly lifted his head up and exclaimed, "I'm concerned about Alina's weight! I think she might be losing weight!" Sean and I looked at each other, and asked Ben if he was worried and why? He responded, "Well, she might lose weight!" I said, "But why would that be a problem, honey?"

Ben looked at me, a little shy, and said, "I just overheard you talking about it, that's all."

"Ben!" I practically yelled, lying down in bed next to him. "You are so awesome to pay attention to what we are saying and overhear that! Yay! We're not worried about Alina's weight, though, honey; we just want her to be healthy. And now that she is eating the way you eat, she will be more healthy!" Ben just smiled.

A bloomin' miracle, as my mother would say.

WEDNESDAY, FEBRUARY 8, 2012

Tough road into friendship

Ben is learning to have friends and to navigate a world of relationships with his peers. He is growing tremendously, with plenty of growing pains in the process. Today, we had a hard day. I did not choose to stay grounded and positive, and was not as helpful as I could have been.

What happened

Ben was exhausted, and seemed to be coming down with a cold or virus, all day long. His WiSH teacher noticed his aberrant behavior in class, and I had noticed in the playroom before school this morning that despite a solid nine to ten hours of sleep, Ben was extremely tired.

After WiSH, four of the boys, including Ben, went outside to play. I was out picking up Alina and returned after they had been out already about forty minutes. Had I been home, I would have brought him in much sooner, since he was fighting a cold. When I arrived,

I saw Ben on a tummy scooter, on his stomach, going slowly down the sidewalk, while the other boys were on upright scooters with helmets on, racing much further down. I went over to talk to the teacher and some other parents, and failed to notice the dynamics taking place among the boys a few hundred yards down the street.

I saw Ben sitting on the sidewalk and became a bit concerned that Ben was fighting a cold and sitting on the cold concrete. I called out for him to come back and that it was time to go in. He didn't respond. I called down again, this time more firmly. Again, he didn't respond. I decided to give it a few more minutes and went back to talking with the other mothers.

Suddenly I heard Ben crying. I looked down toward the children. I listened to see if I had been mistaken in what I heard, but again heard Ben crying, this time more loudly, piteously even. I took off running down the street, and I threw my arms around him. The other boys had run off in the other direction, toward their parents. Ben was crying uncontrollably and saying things I couldn't understand through his tears. He stood up, grabbed the skateboard and purple tummy scooter next to him, and started walking toward home trying to hold the two items rather awkwardly. I gently took them from him and put my arm around him.

When we got back inside, I asked him what had happened. I gradually understood that when the boys went out to play after school, they had gone into the shed and taken out scooters and helmets, but left none for Ben. So he was relegated to the skateboard and tummy scooter, and had to move really slowly, while the other three boys flew down the street on their upright scooters. They left Ben in the dust. Moreover, I found out later from one of the boys that one of the friends had teased Ben about going so slowly, which pushed Ben over the edge.

Ben told me he felt totally left behind and left out of the group, and that they weren't his friends anymore. I tried saying that sometimes friends make mistakes, and they probably were just having so much fun on their scooters—which he was very generous and loving to share with them, along with his helmets—that they just forgot to look out for him. It wasn't right, and it was thoughtless—"Yes, it was!" replied Ben—but it probably wasn't meant to hurt him, since they do love him very much. It was an unloving act, to be sure, but even friends make mistakes sometimes. I shared with him that Mommy and Daddy make a lot of mistakes and apologize to each other when we hurt each other with our mistakes, but we are still best friends. Alina volunteered an example of when her best friend did something that was very mean, and Alina still had her for a best friend anyway.

Ben basically went into a tantruming fit for the next two hours. He yelled, "My friends are now my enemies!" I did everything I could, but I did not bring my best self to the table. I got angry at one point: at him, at myself for not being able to help him, and once again at autism. Life and friends do awful things to us. That's a given; having a neurological overload and meltdown in response to a sock in the gut as a result of an impaired immune system—well, that just didn't seem fair to me this afternoon.

I don't know who had a bigger temper tantrum, Ben or me!

At one point, Ben bit Alina on her arm, and I lost it. I hollered at Ben and would probably have yelled more, but our housemate came in to see what all the upset was, and his presence reminded me that I was supposed to model serenity and reasonableness. So I snapped back at that point and did better. But I did not stay happy, not at all.

I didn't "choose happiness" today. I chose self-pity and anger about the Waldorf school and autism and life not going the way I wanted it to.

Our housemate said to me, "Still, Susan, you have a really great life!" I nearly decked him.

Sean came home at dinnertime and immediately went upstairs with Ben. Ben had wanted some present, a toy or a treat or something, to alleviate some of the pain of the day. He asked for computer time, which makes his autism worse, and I gave it to him, which was not a healthy choice for him. He was online while I bathed Alina, for about twenty-plus minutes, and he stayed very tense afterwards. When Alina and I rejoined him, he was pitching a fit about the video game not working right.

Ben is growing, changing, and hurting as he learns about friendships. Once you have friends, you get hurt. Then you live through it, and the friendship means more. So here's to a young boy's evolution, and a mother doing her best and feeling like she's failing—even when she's not.

THURSDAY, FEBRUARY 9, 2012

At 4:20 this morning, Ben woke me up to tell me, "Mommy, I have to tell you something! I have to tell Elliot I'm sorry!" "Oh really?" I replied, from out of my dreams. "Why?" "Because I called him Meany Elliot yesterday!"

I grinned ear to ear. Yesterday, when he felt hurt, they were his enemies. This morning, after a night of processing and sharing his feelings, they were his buddies again, and he knew he had some amends to make for his part. He had forgiven them for leaving him the dust yesterday afternoon, had truly let go of his hurt and anger, and was now able to look at his own behavior.

FRIDAY, FEBRUARY 10, 2012

Imaginary classmates

It is interesting and noteworthy to me that ever since we began our Son-Rise Program in early 2009, from the moment Ben began to interact with me in the playroom, the focus and theme of most of his stories, isms, and imaginings has been school classes. Ben has created umpteen imaginary classes of animals, children, aliens, and even grown-ups—classes, classes, and more classes. Gee, where do you think he wants to be?

He wants to be in a school with other children, but can't be, so he creates imaginary schools with imaginary children. He wants to have adventures, but can't yet, so he creates imaginary adventures. He loves his family more than anything, so he focuses endlessly on imaginary versions of our family.

So the positive side is that Ben is a brilliant innovator, who never stops creating solutions to resolve his personal wants. On the challenging side, Ben is unwilling (unable?) much of the time to discontinue his imaginary world and focus on the present context. His choice to focus on fantasy rather than reality creates meaningful problems in his friendships with peers, who find his obsession with imaginary stories and characters laughable.

When we were in the process of preparing this year's application to the Waldorf school, I explained to Ben that once he was in school, and particularly during his visit to the school, he needed to reserve imaginary topics for recess or, better yet, for just inside his Son-Rise Playroom. After that, he stopped telling stories at inappropriate times to a significant degree. Then, when Waldorf pulled the rug out from under us a second time, he reverted to a constant focus on imaginary beings and stories.

Ben seems to use imaginary stuff to create the world he wants, that is, a group of school friends, of which he is a member. I wonder if, should he enter an actual community of peers, his obsession with imaginary peers would disappear, or at least substantially decrease. I think it would. I frankly think he's somewhat bored and understimulated, and that he has nothing to do but create imaginary worlds. He also, I believe, associates his playroom with his experience of generating endless imaginary creations and defaults to that mode whenever he is in there. And of course all of us, his Son-Rise Program facilitators, support and celebrate that creativity in the room.

So if he were to go to school next fall, would he emerge from that imaginary focus or would he fall apart? I don't know the answer. We need to get some sort of objective assessment before we can even apply anywhere, so that's the next step.

SUNDAY, FEBRUARY 12, 2012

I had a video feedback with my Son-Rise Program teacher this afternoon. I had sent him six videos of Ben in various situations, including four in his Son-Rise Program playroom. After reviewing the videos, my teacher's opinion was that Ben is not bored, but rather that he is showing autistic behaviors: rigidity, lack of eye contact, and a lack of interest in others, except insofar as they are sources of entertainment for him.

He advised me to go back to basics, with joining, waiting for the green light, celebrating the green light, slowly building, and eventually challenging once interaction was strongly established. He commented, "You know how to do all that." I certainly do. After three years, yes, I do know the basics. And here we are again.

I have been having brat attacks, fits of anger when the children are disobedient toward me or Sean or fighting with one another. This is aberrant behavior for me; I rarely get mad at them. But this week I must have gotten angry—really angry—at them, at least three, if not four, times. I am bottled up. I am angry. I don't want to be here. I am sick of this lifestyle, with people living here and no privacy for Sean and me. I am tired of being caught in a financial stranglehold by spending so much money over the years, despite never taking a real vacation for ourselves over the past five years. I want to feel sorry for myself, because

I want to have a family that can travel, go skiing, go away with other families, and be part of a community of families. We stick our toes in, we get a little of that, but it's still impossible because of Ben's autism.

My teacher and I talked about acceptance. I talked about honesty and not pretending things are okay inside of me when they're not. I need to share more, I need to discuss my challenges and rough feelings, the depth of my fears, and the costs of what we do. We do the right thing, which is to do everything we can to be good parents to Ben and Alina. I do it all for me; it isn't for them alone. I love them, and I want them to be happy and have a great life. I have Sean, I have my parents, I have my support groups, my friends, and my home. I have my health, and I get to be alive and try to live with God.

So we are back to basics, once again. There are worse places to be. There are places, and I have been there, where hope is nowhere to be found. We are still hopeful. What I am lacking, however, and have been constantly lacking lately, is *patience*.

MONDAY, FEBRUARY 27, 2012

This morning Ben and I had the coolest conversation. I am grateful our Son-Rise Program has taught me to question my own assumptions and, most importantly, to ask questions. I asked him, "Ben, sometimes I wonder if you make up imaginary friends because you aren't in school. I think sometimes that if you had more real friends, maybe you wouldn't make up so many imaginary friends. Is that true?" At first he made his face sad and said, "Yes." But two seconds later, he straightened out his face and said, "But I'm not lonely." Then he paused. "I don't do it because I'm lonely! It's just fun!"

Ben is a good teacher for me. He's happy in himself and makes choices that serve him, not for the sake of others or in response to the lack of others.

SUNDAY, MARCH 25, 2012

We have decided to have Alina leave the Waldorf school and be in WiSH. Ben decided it was okay. We also have started the GAPS diet, which is being used by families all over the world to heal their children's autism. Alina is also on GAPS to help her stomach problems.

SATURDAY, MARCH 31, 2012

We had a mini-Seder tonight. Alina read the Four Questions, and we all answered the questions. They both really know the story; I am very pleased. Then we went through the whole Passover story, and I asked them questions throughout. It was highly interactive and exciting to do as a family.

Ben was upset, however, by the killing of the firstborn Egyptian in the Exodus story. He actually wept and asked me, "Do you think they could find any way to bring back their children?" Increasingly upset, he proclaimed, "If my child died, I would kill my other children and myself, so we could all be together again!" Despite my initial horror at the prospect of my son perpetrating a murder-suicide, I saw that Ben was trying to create a resolution to an emotionally intolerable concept—losing a child.

Ben is excited about someday becoming a daddy and actually announced last week—several times—that he wants to have a boy, so the child can carry on the name of Levin and it won't be lost. But Ben's emotions were almost unbearable to him this evening, and that's the way it's been for two days. On a dime he is crying, then laughing again shortly after. It's an emotional roller coaster.

I got into some impatience and frustration today over all of this. Sean asked me, "Why are you letting Ben's sadness make you sad?" Great question. I just want a guarantee that this is really die-off, and not just more autism.

Why am I fighting the idea of Ben's being autistic? He is my child, and he might be autistic to some degree for the rest of his life. Can I accept that? If I can, then I am in a win-win position. Either he recovers, and I am happy, or he doesn't, and I accept him and love him, and I have peace.

We've been on GAPS Intro Diet Stage One for six weeks now, and I just want to be able to give the children something other than broth, soup, fats, boiled meat, poultry, veggies, and sauerkraut juice. I thought we would be beyond this stage by now, and I really start to feel sorry for myself. But I would rather choose to let go of this impatience.

It's just, well . . . we had meatballs for an *afikomen* tonight, for goodness sakes!

SATURDAY, APRIL 14, 2012

I called from Washington, DC last night (Alina and I were there for four days for Passover with my parents), and when I said, "Ben, I love you, babes," he responded, "I love you, too. Bye!" He was so casual. Like saying, "I love you, too" was a nonevent. A casually heart-stopping miracle is what it was! I'll never get over it.

When I got home from DC this afternoon, he said, "You are going to sit and hug me for the rest of the day." *No problem!*

Later, Alina was sitting on the couch looking a little down, and Ben asked, "Alina, do you feel okay?" Again, so casually asked, tone so even and relaxed, and his timing so "normal." Pardon the adjective, but it feels pretty exciting when things feel that way.

Ben then told Alina she should sleep with Daddy, because he thinks Daddy must have missed Alina, ". . . and I think that is true because I felt that way for Mommy!"

THURSDAY, APRIL 19, 2012

Ben went wild at bedtime tonight because he wanted to keep reading, and it was time for bed. I felt a little rigid myself, because I'm concerned his nighttime book choices are stimulating and not restful.

I can't believe I am even worried about something so unimportant when Ben is doing so well.

In any case, he burst into tears and said, "I'm going to be wild until you let me read!" He then kicked, flailed, and bit Sean (not very hard; more symbolic than hurtful). After the whole thing resolved, I let him know there would be consequences tomorrow for his behavior and that I was going to have to think about what was appropriate. He offered that a good consequence would be an extra lesson. I agreed, as lessons are challenging for him.

I went downstairs after kissing the children good night. About five minutes later, I heard Ben's footsteps on the stairs. He came in, looking sheepish. He said Daddy had suggested he apologize to me and that he had asked Daddy if he would get a punishment if he didn't apologize. Daddy had said no and that Ben should only apologize if he wanted to. Ben told me he came down anyway. He asked me, "Can you understand how I was feeling, that I was nervous about getting another punishment?" I replied yes, and that I appreciated very much that he came down to apologize.

I then asked him if he could understand how I felt when he was being so wild and violent. He said yes, and that as a consequence maybe we should be a "bookless house" and I should never take him and Alina to the library again. I laughed and said I thought that was a bad idea and that of course we would still have books. I added that I wanted to give him some books that are good for nighttime, and we could look at them together tomorrow. I then asked if he understood why acting the way he did was not good, and he said, "Yes, because it makes other people crazy." "Yes," I agreed, "and also because you can hurt people." I told him how proud I was of him and kissed him good night.

SUNDAY, APRIL 29, 2012

Ben is making jokes! They are *terrible*, but they are intentional attempts at humor, followed up usually with the questions, "Is that funny? Do you understand my joke?"

It's a great leap from the totally literal and rigid paradigm in which a "typical" autistic person exists.

Ben's main ism is still storytelling. He lives in a world of imagination, peopled with children, teachers, and animals (his three favorite beings on earth next to me and Sean). His stories are endless, often interwoven with each other, wildly imaginative, and extremely consistent. Teachers and students are based on people in Ben's life or on characters in books he's read. Lately he has been developing a particular story line that I find so remarkable that I have been considering looking for a children's book illustrator and setting it all down in print. Tonight after dinner, he asked me if he could read something to me. I was delighted, and even more so when I heard the content.

Ben had written down a summary of the very story I want to do something with!

"The Muffin Monster"

Introduction

Hi my name is Jessica. I'm in Ms Eckel's class. Our computers our [sic] magic. All we have to do is print a picture and put a car on the paper, and then we are in the picture. We have a weird class. Ms. Eckel makes us take challenges in picture world for five hours. And the only way to go back to the real world is to sing the words, "Computers are made up." Instead of learning normally, one day my team learned to make muffins. Come see how we discovered a muffin napper!

Last week in Ben's Son-Rise Program playroom, we spent time going on these "challenges" and having great and wild adventures with the characters from the story.

MONDAY, APRIL 30, 2012

Today we started Stage 3 of the GAPS Intro Diet. The children each had one measly little pancake—those poor little guys! It was as if they were eating pheasant under glass. The pancakes are actually home-made, raw almond butter, grated and drained zucchini, and egg yolks. They loved them! Fried in ghee. Amazing. Tomorrow we will have one pancake in the morning and one in the afternoon.

WEDNESDAY, MAY 2, 2012

This just happened:

Ben: Mommy, when is our next vacation?

Me: Hmm, I'm not sure, BenBen. I know we will definitely be going to the mountains for vacation in July.

Ben: Can we go on one before then?

Me: Well, actually I was thinking we might go somewhere this month, and if you want to help me plan it, we could try and do that! Why are you asking; is there somewhere in particular you want to go?

Ben: Well, I really miss that little boy I met when we were at Grandma and Grandpa's house last time. When Daddy took me to the park then, I met a little boy and I really liked him. I really want to make some friends.

Me: Hmm, Ben. Well, here's the thing. It's actually a little hard to stay friends with people you meet on vacation, because you only meet them there, and you don't have the chance to play with them after the vacation. The really best way to make friends is actually by taking a class, because then you see each other each week, and you like the same things because you're in the same class together. And actually I've been looking for classes for both you and Alina. Would you like to hear about some of the classes that are around here?

Ben: Yeah!

Me: Well, there's a book-writing class in Gloucester that I read about. It's a camp where you go and write stories with other kids, and then you get to make them into real books! And then there are other ones, too.

Ben: The book-writing one is the one for me!

Me: Then that is the one you shall do!

Whose child is this, again?

Then tonight:

Ben: Mommy, I want you to tell me you're proud of me!

Me: Ben, I'm always proud of you. What specifically are you talking about right now?

Ben: Because I tried to help Gavin [Ben's imaginary best friend] find his stuffed animal when he lost it!

Me: Oh Ben, I am so proud of you for that! You are such a great friend to try and help him find it.

Ben: But I could have just made it so he didn't lose it in the first place.

Me: YES! Because you are in control of your imagination, right?

Ben: Yes!

Me: Well, next time you can do that! Great job, Ben!

Ben is starting to understand that he controls his imaginary universe.

Benworld

Ben told me today about "Benworld." It's his world of imagination, where all his imaginary friends, characters, and stories reside. He also told us tonight that everyone has a world like that for themselves.

Alinaworld, Susanworld, Seanworld. Sean told him his world of imagination (Sean's, that is, Seanworld) actually has real people in it, namely Mommy, Ben, and Alina. "But they're not imaginary!" exclaimed Ben. Sean explained that when he is at work all day, in his mind he imagines he is home with us. Ben replied, "So your imaginary world is freedom."

More mistakes

Last week, Ben bit Alina, and I completely lost it. I grabbed him, screaming, *"What is wrong with you? How can you hurt your sister like that? God!"* and threw him onto the couch. It was an awful morning. I felt terrible about myself and at the end of my rope. We are having problems with reactions to certain foods again, and I am responding with fear and rage.

Ben also felt remorseful about his behavior. He bit Alina on Friday, and on Saturday we went to a May Fair with our Waldorf-homeschooling community. Unfortunately, and this was just an error in how the thing was put together, he was not allowed to be in a dance around the maypole that some of the children in a co-op had prepared, and he felt totally rejected.

He said to me that evening, "This was a terrible day. I think God gave me a bad day today because He thought I deserved it." "Because you bit Alina yesterday?" I asked. "Yes."

I told Ben I don't believe God punishes us. Actually, I told him, it's God who gets us through the bad stuff. The bad stuff, I told him, is just life, and everybody has to deal with the bad parts of life from time to time.

I think he believed me. At least he believed that I believed what I was saying. I actually do believe what I was saying and that is why I can survive and embrace this world and all of its difficulties.

F'd up, burned out, need a break

This weekend I felt scared, useless, depressed, despondent, tired, physically in pain, and brain-dead. The ups and downs of this emotional roller coaster are too much for me.

I still feel hopeful. I just feel absolutely, 100 percent shot. Nothing left.

TUESDAY, MAY 8, 2012

My attitude is way, way off. I am angry: at Ben, at myself, and at our situation. I have always believed in a benevolent universe. I still believe it, but I'm angry that Ben has been treated badly—by schools and their administration, by other children, and by unthinking parents who don't realize the harm their actions can cause other people's children.

I wish I could be with other Son-Rise Program families, who understand what it's like to feel self-pity and loss when you hear about little league, Hebrew school, and karate lessons.

What I really want is to let go of this self-pity. I need rest. I think that will help.

WEDNESDAY, MAY 9, 2012

Tonight Ben did something he has never done before quite in this way. The four of us were lying in bed together, snuggling and doing our nighttime routine of prayers, singing, and kisses. Alina fell asleep before singing, so Sean and I sang to Ben alone. We've been singing the same sequence of songs for years and years to the children. We start with *Michael Row*, then *Mockingbird*, then *Baa, Baa, Black Sheep*. Every night, for years and years.

Tonight, as we were singing *Michael Row*, Ben softly began to sing along with us. Sean's eyes bugged out, and he gestured wildly to me. (Ben's back was to him.) I nearly burst into tears. It's not like Ben hasn't been interactive, expressive, and loving with us for a couple of years now. But there was just something about his joining in tonight—especially after the strongly autistic behaviors we've been seeing since Friday—that we both recognized as meaningful.

It was a nice way to end our day. I try to remember that each day and every moment with each other is a gift. I called Sean at work today and asked, "What's *wrong* with me? Why am I choosing such negativity?" Sean replied, "You've gotten too attached to the outcome again. You need to let go."

My husband knows me so well.

SUNDAY, MAY 13, 2012

This was what Ben wrote to me in a card made of a piece of purple construction paper, about 12" by 3". His handwriting, usually pretty good, was indecipherable, so I asked him to read it to me, which he did:

"Dear Mommy, Happy Mother's Day. I love you more than anything. Your the greatest. Nobody is more beautiful than you. Your always right. Ben."

Darn wonderful.

Then this afternoon, I had a great hour in the playroom with Ben and Alina. I brought in a really fun game, complete with song sheets for the song "Witch Doctor" (as in, "Oo, eee, oo aah aah, ting tang, walla walla bing bang . . .") and an obstacle course with three stations. Ben shut me down pretty quickly, despite some pretty gosh-big energy, excitement, and enthusiasm.

Me: Ben, I'm SO excited to play this game with you! [Singing Witch Doctor at the top of my lungs; dancing around the room]

Ben: NO. I don't want to play that game. It's boring.

Me: Great! Thank you for telling me what you think! I'm just going to play it for a while, because it's SOOOOO FUN!! Oo, eee, oo ahh ahh—

Ben: It's boring.

Me: Great! So I'd love to play your game!

Ben: Okay! [Goes to get out plastic animals and blocks]

Me: And then maybe we can play my game after!

Ben: No.

Me: Okay!

It was an awesome session, because *I* had fun. I continued to weave my game, or at least parts of it, into his game, and Ben even started singing the chorus to Witch Doctor at one point. But mostly we played his game, and I made sure I was moving; animating my body, voice, and face; not staying in one place; and really hamming it up. Alina had a Day-Glo-green bathing cap in there for some reason, and I kept putting it on over my eyes and yelling, "Who turned off the lights? What's going on in here? Someone call the police!" and the children were laughing and laughing. It was all very fun.

Then after playroom and before dinner, Ben got really inflexible with Alina, and things began to escalate. Unfortunately, in response, I became tense and inflexible myself. Ben wanted a sticker in one of Alina's sticker books (which has about fifty stickers in it), and Alina didn't want to share. Ben went pretty crazy, and I could see another bite situation in the making. I became self-righteous and preachy toward Ben, which didn't help. I told Alina she was not generous, and I told Ben he was rigid and demanding and couldn't be that way if he wanted to have good relationships. (Oops. Again.)

Then I felt sorry for myself (again), sorry for Sean and me (again), hopeless about Ben (again), and generally negative. Sometimes you just need to stop thinking and talking, and go relax. So I did.

I'm not feeling negative anymore. It's time for bed. It's been a complicated day, but it's also been a good one.

TUESDAY, MAY 15, 2012

Ben got lost for almost an hour today. We had finished indoor recess at WiSH, and Miss Claudine and Alina went outside to plant a raspberry bush. I invited Ben to go out to join in the planting, but he wanted to keep reading his book. I gave him some more time—he requested fifteen minutes—and then he was willing to go outside. He asked where they were, and I told him, "They are on the Foley side of the house, right outside." The Foleys are a family who live up the street from us.

I worked inside for a while, maybe twenty minutes, and then Claudine and Alina came back inside. "I guess Ben never wanted to come out, eh? Is he still reading?" asked Claudine. I looked up, startled. "You mean he's not with you?" Claudine replied, "No, he never came out!"

We spent the next hour searching for Ben. We looked all over the house, around the block, down all the side streets, and down into the woods. An elderly lady came driving by at one point and told us she had seen a little boy waiting for someone to come find him, that he had asked her where his sister and teacher were, and that he was just up the street. But when we ran up the street, Ben wasn't there.

We continued to look for him. I called the police. While we were waiting for the police to arrive, our housemate, Dylan, mentioned that he had seen Ben on a bike ride going toward a house on our street a day or so ago, and Dylan had just assumed there was a friend who lived there or something. As soon as Dylan mentioned that, I realized where Ben was. The driveway to the Foleys' house actually leads to a path down into the woods behind our house, and Claudine had taken the children there during WiSH a bunch of times. I realized Ben must have gone down there. Claudine immediately set off on Sean's bike to see if Ben was there, and by that time, happily, our au pair, Florian ("Flo"), had discovered Ben near that same area, lost in the woods behind the Foleys' house.

The police arrived about fifteen minutes after I called them, just in time to see Ben and Flo walking back toward our house.

It was terrifying. As a parent, you visualize the most horrible things. While Ben was still lost, Alina also thought it would be a great idea to mention the missing child poster at our gymnastics studio—at which point I nearly threw up.

The miraculous contrast

As I mentioned, the police arrived right before Ben did and were asking me questions. I still didn't know what had happened, so I wasn't saying much.

When Ben got to us, however, he voluntarily explained what had, in fact, happened. He said, "Mommy told me to go to the Foley side house, so I did. But Miss Claudine and Alina weren't there! So then I thought, maybe they are in the woods; that's a good place to plant a raspberry bush. So I went down into the woods behind the Foleys' house, but I couldn't find them. And then I got lost."

"Oh Ben!" I cried. "You are so brave! That was so smart to check for them in the woods, and I am so sorry I gave such confusing instructions! Were you scared when you got lost, poor baby?" "Yes," Ben said, "It was scary." I hugged him and hugged him, and then we said goodbye to the police and went inside. Then Alina left for swimming, and Ben and I sat on the couch and rested.

Ben was exhausted and wanted to read. While he was reading, Sean called (I hadn't called him, so he didn't know what had happened), and as I was telling him about all of it, Ben took the phone from me and proceeded to tell Sean, *blow by blow*, what had happened. He was expressive, honest, and accurate.

Like I said, Ben used to bolt all the time, but it was instinctive, sensory-driven, and impulsive. He wanted to run, so he ran, with no thought of the impact on others. But today, his venture into the woods was motivated by his desire to follow his mother's instructions and to be obedient. His eventual rescue was joyful to him because he returned to his family and friends.

Moreover, today Ben went *strategically* and *logically* into the woods. He misinterpreted my unfortunately ambiguous instructions about the Foleys' house and wound up in a location where he couldn't find his teacher and his sister. He made a logical guess, based on reasonable assumptions (plants grow in woods; maybe they are planting the raspberry bush in the woods), and went into the woods to find them. He got lost, he felt scared, he asked someone for help (the elderly lady in the car), and he responded with joy and relief when our au pair finally found him.

Then he told his daddy all about what had happened. Then this evening he hugged me, told me he had had a terrible day, that he had been very scared, and asked if he could sleep in our bed tonight.

TUESDAY, MAY 15, 2012

Every morning, the children and I take either a morning walk or a morning bike ride. Afterward we come in, and the children write in their journals. Alina, at seven, copies some words I give her or draws a picture I suggest. It's beautiful. Ben, at nine, I have instructed to observe at least three things during our outside time to put into his journal.

Today, Ben wrote, "I saw a man, Red Rover and a curve in the road," and drew a picture of a rose bush.

Beauty and innocence.

FRIDAY, MAY 18, 2012

More of Ben's journal entries
I played baseball today 23 [his number of home runs so far].

I did 65 jumps today at the jump rope. I road my bike all the way up the hill. Today I evan [sic] made meat balls with Dylan. I learned to knit.

It is all true. Ben is on his third day of knitting. He is experiencing life, and his world is expanding, little by digestible bit at a time. We had a playdate yesterday with a little boy, a friend who was in WiSH until Ben, in a state of GAPS-induced yeast withdrawal, bit him, and his parents understandably withdrew the boy from the program. The mother told me her sons had a great time with Ben and Alina yesterday, and they were here for hours. Today we had an activity planned, and Ben wanted to stay home and do playroom time instead. I celebrated him for taking care of himself and embraced some much-needed mother-and-daughter time for me and Alina.

Ben had a wonderful few hours in the playroom and even a second bike ride. Also, he told me when Alina and I arrived home at dinnertime, "Mommy, I have some bad news. I think I'm coming down with a cold." He has indeed been sneezing for two days and is now slightly cold-y. He intuitively knew the best place for him to be was home today and not out with a bunch of kids! I'm learning to listen to my children when they communicate their needs. I don't always give them what they want, but I'm trying to listen and consider what they say.

I love the line, "I saw a man, Red Rover and a curve in the road."

FRIDAY, MAY 18, 2012

Ben's journaling continues

I saw a mailbox, in a flower basket. And sparkles on the sidewalk and a clip on a mailbox on my bike ride.

Today I saw a rocky hill, leaves and buttercup.

SUNDAY, MAY 20, 2012

I've decided to go my parents' house for a few days to rest. I have set up the schedule for the week (homeschool, Ben's Son-Rise Program, this au pair here, this housemate there, this one's taking Alina to gymnastics at such-and-such time, etc.). Going away for any period of time, as a homemaker, is an exhausting proposition. Add in special needs, special foods, and a Son-Rise Program, and you may as well not even go.

But I am going. The schedule is done, my bags are packed, and I am ready.

Ben is in great shape right now: responsive, interested, present, and working hard. Still somewhat cold-y and a little low energy, but socially strong. He was unable to handle the GAPS Intro Stage 3 foods, so he is still on GAPS Intro Stage 2, and that's where we're staying until I return from my getaway.

At dinner, I said to Ben, "I'm going to really miss you this week, sweetheart." I said this with no expectation of response, because I've learned not to invite disappointment. But to my delight, Ben replied, without a blink, "Yeah, I'm going to miss you, too, Mommy. It's going to be like a nightmare not being able to see you."

What a nice bon voyage.

Chapter 5
Conversations and Connections

*B*en and I were sitting together this evening, when suddenly he blurted out, "I feel like I've had a miserable childhood."

BAM. Didn't see that one coming.

Me: You do, Ben?

Ben: Yes.

Me: I always thought you were happy, Ben. You weren't happy?

Ben: I always felt like I was out of the ordinary. Everywhere I was.

Me: Do you still feel that way? Even at temple, for example?

Ben: No. There I have friends.

He sat and looked at me.

My eyes filled with tears. Ben looked disturbed and asked me, "Mom? Why the eyes?" I told him it was hard for me to hear that he had been unhappy. "Well," he said, "maybe only a quarter unhappy?"

Later we talked about other children whom we know, who also have it hard. Two of his classmates come from orphanages. One never knew her parents, and the other knew them and they couldn't keep her. Another classmate lost her father when she was four years old. "And you had a hard childhood, too," Ben pointed out, referring to the death of my older brother when we were teenagers. "Yes, Ben, but I wouldn't say I didn't have a happy childhood, because I did. It was just hard, too."

At the end of our conversation, I said to Ben, "I love getting to know you, talking to you, and having these times with you." I continued, "Before I couldn't reach you at all, but now I am really getting to know you. And Alina and you are both so thoughtful and interesting." I really am "meeting" both of them more and more, all the time.

It's startling, that one can give birth to children, raise them, be with them constantly, love them, care for them, and yet only know a small part of who they are, what they feel and believe, and what fills their minds. There is a gap between grown-ups and children, a necessary gap, but a gap nonetheless. With our conversation tonight, I felt like Ben and I bridged a bit of that gap.

Later I kissed Ben good night, after prayers, and he grinned at me. I think we both enjoyed our talk.

LIFE IN NEW YORK

In June 2012, after reluctantly accepting that the best educational environment for Ben was homeschool, I suddenly discovered the Otto Specht School (OSS), a school just outside of New York City that uses a Waldorf curriculum in an environment designed to support children with varying types of learning disabilities.

Otto Specht appeared to have everything we wanted in a school for Ben. The only problem was that it was located in New York. Thrilled at the thought of actually finding a school with a Waldorf curriculum that could work for Ben, but frightened at the prospect of such a radical relocation, Sean and I drove the following week to New York to meet with the school director. Once we saw the school, it felt right, but we didn't know if they would accept him. After all of the previous rejections, we were afraid. We applied to the school, and two weeks later, the director called to tell us they had accepted Ben. Moreover, that same week, we received notice that the local mainstream Waldorf school, Green Meadow Waldorf, located just around the corner from Otto Specht, had accepted Alina into its fall class as well.

So, in a wild and unexpected turn of events, in September 2012, we moved to New York so that Ben could start his next school year at Otto Specht—a real Waldorf school.[†]

In reaction to our decision, our parents, extended family, and closest friends seriously questioned our judgment. The risk was huge, but I was as clear about OSS as I had been about Ben's Son-Rise Program when I discovered it years earlier and announced to Sean that I wanted to withdraw Ben from kindergarten. Over the course of my Son-Rise Program years, I had learned to trust my instincts and my intuition. I wanted a Waldorf education for Ben, because my instincts told me that it would be the most effective and healing education for him.

Even louder than my instincts was Ben's voice in my ears: "I want to go to a real school, Mommy." If no "real" Waldorf schools in Boston would accept Ben, and there was a "real" Waldorf school in New York that was designed for children with special needs, then we had to go. In a wonderful further turn of events, Sean's employer offered to let Sean telecommute from New York to Boston—although he would need to actually commute to Boston and be away from the family for two weeks out of every month. But he could keep his job and his pension. Doors were opening.

---

[*]   Green Meadow Waldorf School is one of the nation's oldest and most well-established Waldorf schools.

[†]   Otto Specht was a German doctor who started life as an autistic child, and who was the first-ever student of Rudolf Steiner, the polymath founder of Waldorf curriculum, biodynamic farming, and Anthroposophy, a "spiritual science." Otto's parents hired Steiner to work with him when Otto was a child. After a number of years working with Steiner, Otto recovered sufficiently to go to a regular school, and later went on to become a medical doctor.

So we rented out our home in Boston, found a place to live for a year in Chestnut Ridge, packed up our things, and moved—all in three months. After decades in Boston, we were suddenly New Yorkers.

BLOGGING LIFE IN NEW YORK

JUNE 2012

Four weeks ago, our world turned upside down when Sean and I decided to move to New York. Otto Specht is a private, Waldorf-based school for children with learning disabilities, *including autism.*

Sean nearly had a heart attack when I told him about the school, but after he heard the details, he got cautiously onboard. The following week, Sean and I drove to New York and met with the school director. Two weeks later, both children were accepted at their new schools: Ben at Otto Specht and Alina at the Green Meadow Waldorf School, the mainstream school located just moments from Otto Specht.

I am sad that I will not get to homeschool them anymore. I cherish our lesson times together. I am heartbroken to leave Boston. But for Ben to be in school, and for Alina to be in a healthy, established, happy Waldorf environment—it's worth any sacrifice.

THURSDAY, JUNE 21, 2012

We have been on Stages 1 to 3 of the GAPS Introductory Diet for over three months now, which is a long time to be eating nothing but bone broth, boiled meats and vegetables, egg yolks, and ghee or tallow (cooked animal fat). Ben and Alina are unbelievable troupers; they don't complain, and they seem to really enjoy these very limited food choices. But it should not be taking this long.

Accordingly, our GAPS consultant asked Dr. Natasha Campbell-McBride, the Russian doctor who invented GAPS, about Ben's situation. Dr. Campbell-McBride thought it might be parasites. I was horrified. Ben tested negative for parasites years ago, but the tests are notoriously unreliable. So we will be trying CD, chlorine dioxide, a compound that, when activated and ingested, eliminates toxic parasites from the body.

Ben continues to make progress. During our playroom session today, I asked him how he was feeling about school.

Me: Ben, how are you feeling about going to your new school in a couple of months?

Ben: A little scared.

Me: Scared? What are you feeling scared about?

Ben: Well . . . I'm very quiet.

Me: And?

Ben: What if that's not okay, that I'm very quiet?

Me: Ben, it is so wonderful that you can share that fear with me! Why do you think there would be anything wrong with being quiet?

Ben: I don't know.

Me: You know, some people are very quiet, and that's fine. Other people are loud, and that's also fine. You and Daddy are both pretty quiet, which is who you are. Alina and I both talk all the time, and that's who we are. It's really fine. What else are you afraid about?

Ben: What if I do something wrong, and I don't know it?

Me: Sweetheart, whatever you do in school, Otto Specht is a place for children to learn how to be with other children. So if you do something and the teacher wants to teach you a different way, she will. But that's why you're there: to learn! So you don't have to worry at all.

Ben: I think I get it! I think Otto Specht is a school for children who need to learn to be better, and then when they're better they can go to Green Meadow!

Me: Well, I don't think the children need to be "better" exactly. I think they just need to learn how to be with other children, for whatever reason. Or they need to learn how to read or something else that will help them to be better students. The children there have different needs, and that's why they are there. And not all the children would like to go to Green Meadow, because the classes there are enormous. Some of them have as many as thirty children!

Ben: [grinning] I think that would be great, to be in such a big class, because there would be so many chances for friendships!

SUNDAY, JUNE 24, 2012

Over the past six months, Ben has developed a very intelligent and charming sense of humor, which he often expresses through jokes he makes up. Here are just a few:

1. What is imaginary that you put on your face?
   Makeup!
2. What do you call fish that isn't generous?
   Shellfish!
3. What three sports are really boring?
   Snowboring, surfboring, and skateboring!

TUESDAY, JUNE 26, 2012

Sean and I are both exhausted and not sleeping well even when we get to bed on time.

But . . . as I was leaving for a meeting the other night, I called out, "Love you guys!" to the children. Ben responded, quietly, "Love you too!" He has told me he loves me only a handful of times in his life, even since his emergence, and I am still shocked when it happens. I asked him, "Did you just say 'Love you too?'" "Yup!" Ben answered.

THURSDAY, JUNE 28, 2012

Ben is in the playroom now with one of our Son-Rise Program staff. Ben just spent half an hour telling me about the imaginary dog show this Sunday to which he's taking his imaginary puppy, Fluffer (age three, all white). There are eight or nine events and twenty dogs from all over Massachusetts participating. The judge's name is Steve. Some of the dog-show events are an uphill jump-rope contest; a basketball game; an ice hockey game; a baseball game that God has put a spell on so no matter the skill levels, the person with the most recent birthday to the day of the show will win; a gymnastics obstacle course; a skate-boarding race; and a T-ball game.

We had a hilarious conversation. I challenged him about every event, arguing that dogs can't do *this* and dogs can't do *that*. We were both cracking up, and it was so fun. He sat with me the whole time. He didn't get up and down. He gave me uninterrupted eye contact. His sentences were coherent, his replies to my questions timely and contextually appropriate, and he totally got my jokes.

FRIDAY, JULY 6, 2012

My parents were here this past week, because they live in DC and it's a furnace there right now. Some notable events took place:

1. On Wednesday, Ben and my dad had their first real conversation, which lasted over twenty minutes, and then another one the next day. That's a first. Ben's never given my dad the time of day.

2. Yesterday evening, my dad read Ben a story while Ben snuggled with him.

3. Last night, Sean suggested to Ben that he say good night to my mom. Ben walked over to my mom, hugged her, and spontaneously said, "I'm really going to miss you, Grandma."

4. Finally, this morning, when Mom and Dad were leaving, I said, "Hugs all around! Grandma and Grandpa are leaving!" Ben jumped right up—no auditory-processing delay—and gave my dad a big hug, *with arms*, and said, "Bye, Grandpa!"

These things were not happening even three months ago.

One other note: Ben has a sensory tic of putting his finger into his nose constantly. That tic has lessened dramatically this week.

MONDAY, JULY 9, 2012

What a great day. Today was Ben and Alina's first day of story-writing camp. The teacher shared with me this evening, when I called her to check how things went, that she had initially been concerned Ben might not have the stamina for the whole day. "But he kept up with *everything!*" she exclaimed. Ben told me a lot about his day, amazing me. I know many neurotypical nine-year-olds would not choose to do that. He told me about his two new friends, Thomas and Max, who are around the same age as he is. They spent the morning playing getting-to-know-you games and painting pages for their books. Then they ate lunch and played at the beach for two hours, and finally, they assembled the pages of their books.

Ben seemed comfortable, happy, and relaxed. The campers played and worked in a circle, and according to Flo, our au pair, who spent the day with the children at camp, Ben stayed with the group the whole time. Ben fully participated in the games and had no meltdowns or exhaustion afterward.

WEDNESDAY, JULY 11, 2012

Today was the third day of book-writing camp, and both kids are having a *blast*. The camp runs from nine to three every day, including two hours of beach/lunch time. Ben has stayed with *all* of the games, activities, and book-writing projects and has shown no signs of the constant fatigue that in the past would have greatly hindered his capacity to participate in such a long day. We are seeing great gains lately in eye contact, responsiveness, and humor, which I attribute to camel milk and CD, which we started again recently.

Then tonight, the four of us were having a great big love-fest at nigh-nighs, singing and laughing and hugging. Ben suddenly blurted out to Sean, "You're the best present of all, Daddy!" I thought Sean was going to cry. He got quiet and said, "Ben, that's the nicest thing you've ever said to me." Alina, not to be outdone, chimed in, "You're *both* the best presents of all!"

FRIDAY, JULY 13, 2012

This morning Ben asked me when he would be able to have almond-butter-and-honey sandwiches again. I told him I have to watch for reactions to the almond butter, which we are gingerly trying now, one teaspoon a day, to see signs of yeast flare-ups and consequent autistic symptoms. "If I don't see symptoms of autism flaring," I explained, "like not responding to me, not making eye contact, not wanting to play with your peers, then I'll know the almond butter isn't causing problems, and then we can go on to try the sandwiches."

"Or," I added, "like circuiting." Circuiting refers to running around and around with no apparent point of destination. It can be a sensory thing for children with autism.

"Circuiting," I continued, "can be a symptom of autism."

"*Or*," replied Ben, with a big grin on his face, "it can just be a symptom of having *fun*!"

Gotcha, Mommy!

Last night when I tucked Ben into bed, I said, "I love you, Ben!" Ben replied, "And I *loooooooove yooooooooou toooooooooo*!"

Seriously. I'm going to be checked into a mental hospital by the end of the month. These highs and lows are a lot to handle.

SUNDAY, JULY 15, 2012

Sean and I drove to New York this weekend to sign papers on the rental home I found for this coming year. We move September 1. Last night we called the children to say good night, and Alina and Ben both got on the phone. At the end of the call, I said, "I love you, Ben! I love you, Alina!" Alina responded, "I love you too, Mom." Then there was a pause. I said, "Okay, we'll talk to you guys tomorrow." Suddenly Ben blurted out, "Me too! I mean I love you too!"

We got home today. Just now, Ben came downstairs to snuggle a bit on the couch. I can't believe how commonplace it has become for him to snuggle with me, appropriately express love and affection, and easily enter into conversations about interesting and relevant things. So here we were, sitting together, and all of a sudden Ben said, "I have a question. I heard that some people think that you have another life after this one. Is that true?" Apparently Alina had told her brother about reincarnation. Ben and I proceeded to have a conversation about where the soul goes after death. I shared my belief that the body dies, but not the spirit. I told him other people believe different things about the life of the spirit, post-death. It was a fun conversation.

I'm in awe that Ben has matured and developed to a point where we can converse about topics like that. Four years ago, we had no conversations at all, *ever*. I remember being at a Son-Rise Program course and crying at the idea that Ben might someday tell me about something he had done in school that day. Such conversations are frequent today.

We have a long way to go. Ben's speech patterns, in particular (not the content of what he says, but the way he talks), are very different from that of a normal child. He still gets stuck sometimes, rigid around what he wants. He still suffers with mitochondrial dysfunction and low energy.

But he has come a long way. I remember when I used to come home from being away for a couple of days or more and how disappointed—shattered, actually—I would feel when I saw how impaired he was. Coming home today from New York, after being away for two days, I felt the opposite. I felt hopeful, thrilled even, about his progress. We recently introduced camel milk—the only milk Ben can tolerate because it has no casein, the hard-to-digest protein in dairy products, and is healing to the immune system. The camel milk and the CD are having a visible effect.

MONDAY, JULY 16, 2012

Tonight, I said good night to the children, and as always, I said, "I love you!" Alina eked out an "I love you, too, Mama"—she was very tired—and Ben, sitting near me on the bed, looked me *squarely in the eye* and said, firmly, "I love you, too." The other night when he said, "I love you, too," he hadn't looked at me, and so I asked him to say it again, looking at me. He did so, but afterward I felt silly, because I felt I had forced the moment. But tonight I saw that he had really heard me and was, it seemed, deliberately looking right in my eyes to communicate in the way I had requested.

He loves me, he's telling me so, and he's looking in my eyes.

THURSDAY, JULY 19, 2012

Ben has a story idea about time-zone borders. In it, there is a house that is on both sides of the border, so when you walk from one room to another you are in another time zone. He also has another idea about a house on different state or country borders: when you walk from one room to another you are in another state or country. What a mind.

SUNDAY, JULY 29, 2012

Sean and I are both tense, and we had a nasty fight. He's extremely anxious about his new commute between Boston and New York. I'm concerned about him. We're both miserable at the thought of being apart from each other. Between the CD, the new medications, the packing, moving in four weeks, our typical workloads and stress, and dealing with all of the emotions around the massive changes coming up for all of us, life is pretty full-on right now.

TUESDAY, JULY 31, 2012

Two-word love song

This morning Ben ran upstairs and asked me and Sean where a certain paper was. I told him where I thought it was, and he ran down the stairs. Suddenly he stopped, turned around, and yelled out, "Thanks, Mom!"

WEDNESDAY, AUGUST 1, 2012

Day Four of the CD-parasite protocol: Ben's teacher from this past school year visited today and remarked, "He's so *with* us! Wow!"

It's true. He's more responsive, bright, and connected than we've ever seen before.

MONDAY, AUGUST 6, 2012

Note from Sean

For the second time in my life, my son told me he loves me! Ben is nine years old, but, before today, he had only said it once, and that was a few years ago. Please don't get me wrong. I know Ben loves me. He passionately loves me. I think it's been a guy thing, you know . . . guys don't tell guys they love them, although I tell Ben all the time. But I never ask if he loves me nor do I ever look for it.

When I came home from work, Susan told me as part of our move that she had cleaned out a room and asked me what I wanted to do with a book. I told her I wanted to keep it, saying that someone who loves me (Susan) gave it to me. Out of the blue, Ben suddenly exclaimed, "*I love you.*" It was very matter of fact, as if he were saying, "You all knew it; I'm just saying it out loud." Then Ben went back to his book. I was overjoyed.

Is it filling a hole in my heart? Repairing my damaged soul? No. I've known all along that my son loves me. Like I said, it's a guy thing. But Ben had the desire to connect with me and make a loving, caring statement. It was a wonderful example of him thinking of others and having a desire to make a connection.

WEDNESDAY, AUGUST 8, 2014

Small gestures tell me Ben is changing.

Just now, in our bedroom, I was talking to my father on the phone, sitting in my quiet-time chair. Ben, lying in our bed, listening in, chose to get up, carry over an afghan, lay it across my legs, smile, and go back to bed.

He knows I get cold easily.

SUNDAY, AUGUST 12, 2012

This afternoon, Ben said to me, "I have so much stammering, and hesitate so much. I've noticed you never do that, you don't hesitate with your words." I had no idea he knew.

WEDNESDAY, AUGUST 15, 2012

My little humorist

Ben was awake last night, with me, from 3:15 till about 5:30 AM. Dee-lightful. Around 4 AM, he asked, "Do you want to hear a joke I just made up, Mommy?" Nothing better to do, I thought to myself. "I'd *love* to, Ben!" I responded. Big three E's. Ben asked, "Why did the fan leave the baseball game?" "Why, Ben?" "Cause he wanted to hit a home run! Get it?"

I laughed out loud. Life can be good—even at 4 AM.

SUNDAY, AUGUST 19, 2012

Ben was, by turns, today and yesterday, totally off-the-wall with hysteria and tears and then presenting with moments of radical lucidity. Definitely going through something.

TUESDAY, AUGUST 21, 2012

Ben has been somewhat remote for the past two days, not responding to questions or calls, very diminished eye contact, and generally not as connected as he was a few days ago. Likely causes:

1. He tried ham (totally clean, from our beloved Amish farm; but still, it's pork) the day before yesterday and went crazy for it. Always a bad sign, especially when followed by autistic symptoms like we are currently seeing.

2. He is experiencing a lot of trepidation about our imminent move (ten days and counting!) and all that it represents. Loss of home, loss of Daddy two weeks a month, loss of what he knows and knows he loves, and finally, going to a school where he has to repeat third grade, about which he is very upset. All those feelings may be affecting his ability to connect.

WEDNESDAY, AUGUST 22, 2012

"No you are!"

This morning Ben did something with me he has never done before. He was about to go on a morning walk, and he said, "I need someone to watch my game so it doesn't get messed up while I'm gone." "I'll watch it," I volunteered. "Thanks, Mommy. You're the *best*!" Ben exclaimed. "Well," I replied, "I think *you're* the best, Ben!"

Ben then grinned and said, "No, *you* are!"

I replied, also grinning, "No, *you* are!"

Ben replied, "*You* are!"

"*You* are!"

"You!"

"You!"

And back and forth three or four more times, laughing with each other. We have never done this together before.

We spent the past two days in what I believe to be a ham-induced fog (no more smoked food for us), and now today, having processed it out of his system, he is completely interactive and present with us. Amazing.

"No, you are!"

TUESDAY, AUGUST 28, 2012

This morning, Ben wrote a letter to his friend, Robbie, who got hurt yesterday in a soccer game. He clearly needs help with punctuation and capitalization, but boy, he loves his friends:

Dear Robbie Im sorry you got an ingerie. Its really sad Does Tristen know about it? Would you like to play Hospital with me? Did your Mom Make Sure You dont Have inguries Anywhere else? Im asking these questions to cheer you up Ben

PS Even though you got hurt dont hurt Anyone else

FRIDAY, AUGUST 31, 2012

Today I asked Ben why he was not answering me when I asked him stuff—to join us for lunch, to clean up, whatever. "Is it a reaction to the apples, honey?" I asked. "Is that why you're not responding to me?" We recently added in a little bit of apples to see if he could handle it.

"No," Ben replied. "It's just a bad attitude."

WEDNESDAY, SEPTEMBER 5, 2012

We have arrived! We're here in New York now and so far, so good. Both children are excited. It doesn't feel like home to me, but as Sean reminded me, beginnings are hard. Unfortunately, this week I made an error and tried to give Ben some foods he is not ready for. For those of you who are parents, imagine not being able to give your child anything besides broth, boiled vegetables, boiled meats, fats, and pancakes made with ground chicken, eggs, and broth. So even though he didn't request it, I gave him some fresh fruit (apples and pears, in small amounts), and I made a meatloaf with ground turkey and tomato paste. He loved all of it, and couldn't get enough. I wanted so badly for him to be able to have these things. My creativity for imagining new versions of broth is just at a low ebb right now.

As a result, Ben zoned out. We lost responsiveness and eye contact. Granted, he's exhausted and probably a bit bored. But I know autism when I see it. He stops being interested in us, and his flexibility plummets.

Ben came in today, and I asked him how he thought he was doing with the fruit and the meatloaf. He said, "Can I cheat and say I'm fine? Even when I know I'm reacting to them? Do people do that?" I told him he *can* say he's fine, but I actually want to know the truth so that I can give him the foods that are healing to him and that won't cause autism. I asked him if he noticed a feeling that he wanted to do some autism, and he said, "Yes," without batting an eye.

I told him that we will be staying away from the fruit and meatloaf for a while. I said, "I truly believe that you will heal enough at some point to be able to eat some more of the foods you love, sweetheart." Ben asked me, "How do you know?" I replied, "Because you are healing, and as you heal your tummy, you'll be able to handle much more."

Ben is needy right now and wants endless kisses and hugs. Today he needed a little nap, and as I was tucking him in, he pulled me to him and said, "You take my breath away." How does one describe how it feels to be so deeply loved, after years of being utterly unseen by the same child who now loves you so fervently?

FRIDAY, SEPTEMBER 7, 2012

When I asked Ben today how he was feeling about school starting on Monday, he said, "A little nervous, but I know I'm going to have fun, too." When Sean arrived from Boston this evening, Ben repeated that he was nervous about Monday and then added, "But I'm looking forward to it, too."

Tonight we went to a cookout at Ben's school, and Sean, Alina, and I all had a pleasant evening. But the biggest thrill was Ben, who was, and I'm not exaggerating, *downright gregarious*. He spoke to people whom he had never met before, he conversed comfortably with his teachers, and he participated in the games the children played after dinner. This year is going to bring a lot of miracles. I feel affirmed and confirmed in our decision, and after this helluva week, I am very grateful for that reassurance! We are in God's hands.

MONDAY, SEPTEMBER 10, 2012

Ben's first day at Otto Specht

We started our Son-Rise Program in December '08, at which point we took Ben out of kindergarten, so today was Ben's first day of school in four years.

At 8:30, I drove over to the school with Ben. Sean met us there. We met his teacher and the other children in his class—three adorable girls, all Ben's age. We had a circle with the other elementary-age children at the school, where we all introduced ourselves. Ben said, "I'm Ben," right on cue. At one point, he tried to respond to something the teacher had said, but he couldn't find his words and stammered the same introductory phrase over and over again. But it was okay.

Then we walked down a road to another building, where the teachers of the school presented an assembly that was welcoming and beautiful, and into which they had clearly invested substantial time, energy, and love. The director of the school introduced the children, class by class. Thankfully, Ben stood at the right moment as she presented his class.

The school director presented several brief commentaries on various aspects of the school and introduced some of the teachers.

Ben's response to it all was both anxiety provoking and thrilling. Ben, having been out of school for so long, is not yet aware of assembly etiquette, and emphatically raised his hand with constant questions throughout the twenty-five-minute program. Seated in the front row, Ben waved his hand under the director's nose until she called on him. Or, if she failed to call on him despite his frenetic waving, he simply blurted out his comment or question. Sean and I sweated bullets together as Ben continued to interrupt the proceedings.

Ben stayed engaged the whole morning. His questions, while poorly or ignorantly timed, were intelligent and curious. He asked, for example, what other instruments the piano-playing music teacher played. He burst out dancing during a particularly upbeat song the director and the other teachers presented. He called out, "I want to sing!" when he saw one of the songs on the song sheet. Near the end, he asked about the ending time of the assembly.

He was listening, present, completely involved, and possibly the least autistic person in the room!

At one point, after Ben asked one of his questions, I had a vision of Ben in a college seminar, responding with active, intellectual excitement to some course material. Ben has proven himself to be a critical, rather than a passive, thinker. He doesn't take things at face value, doesn't accept things just because someone says they are a certain way. He thinks for himself. He has an inquisitive, persistent, and eager mind.

For years, all of my visions of Ben's future were dark. I remember one night, when Ben had turned some corner and was a little bit closer to emerging from the autism, I said to Sean, "I think he's graduated to bag boy!" I joked, but my fear was deep. Today I envisioned my son as an excited college student.

He was tired after school, but cheerful. He did two hours in his Son-Rise Program playroom, during which he was manic, with a lot of circuiting. For a first day, he did amazingly well.

We are on the road. I won't say the end is in sight, because we have a long way to go. But the Ben I lovingly watched today was completely different from the Ben we knew before all of our work of the past several years. As I wrote to the school director tonight, words cannot adequately express my gratitude to these people who have accepted my son and, in so doing, have given my family a place to belong.

TUESDAY, SEPTEMBER 11, 2012

Sean just went in to check on Ben; it's late, and he wanted to see if Ben had fallen asleep yet. Sean bent down to kiss Ben. Simultaneously, Ben lifted up his head to kiss Sean, and the two knocked heads. Sean immediately asked, "Are you okay, Ben?" Ben replied, "A little." There was a pause, and then Ben asked Sean, "And you?" Sean was rubbing his own forehead at that moment, and Ben reached up, pulled Sean's hand away, and kissed Sean's head where they had hit each other.

For the millionth time I'll say, for parents who have not known autism, a child knocking a parent's head and then asking if the parent is okay—normal. *In our family—revolutionary.*

Watching Ben at school these past two days, I can't help but compare and contrast him to the other children. Next to them, he seems so impaired, his speech halting and disjointed, his voice high, his words mispronounced (*e.g.,* "dat" for that, and "fank you" for thank you), and his lack of understanding of social cues and rules constantly evident.

But he wants to be there. He is aware of other people and happy to be with them. He is funny; he constantly throws out puns and jokes. He is invested academically; he wants to learn. He is deeply kind; he never fails to express concern about those who seem to be struggling even a little.

I am so proud of him. He is Ben. He is big-hearted, brilliant, beautiful, true, insightful, funny, and sweet. He has had autism, and he still has difficulties. But he is not only finally in the game—he is playing hard, enjoying himself, and showing up courageously.

WEDNESDAY, SEPTEMBER 12, 2012

I am eager to get back to the Son-Rise Program, as our focus has been predominantly Waldorf curriculum, Otto Specht, finding a place to rent and people to rent our Boston house, moving, and the parasite protocol. Not much time for team meetings, observations/feedbacks, developmental-model review, and finding new members. Ben had his third day of school today. They did eurythmy, which is a Steiner-based form of movement therapy, a sort of poetry in motion, and also German! I am in heaven. Up until today, Ben has been doing half days at school to get adjusted.

Tomorrow will be his first full day. I am about to have actual, full days without the children, with time to build games, organize, do team meetings, and zero in once again on Ben's Son-Rise Program. Every day I wonder if the school will contact us to tell us that Ben cannot stay, that he is too impaired, too much of a distraction to the other children, and that they can't help him. Small wonder that I hold this fear, after our earlier rejects. But this school is different and is designed for children who need support.

It might take time for me to trust, but so far things seem to be going okay. Ben is so happy.

THURSDAY, OCTOBER 4, 2012

We miss Daddy when he's in Boston. But the children love their schools. Truly love them. They love their teachers, their friends, and their work. Ben is happier than I have ever seen him. He feels a sense of belonging. He's finally part of a pack and is loved and accepted by everyone there. The Otto Specht children are generally kind, bright, caring, and hyper. I'm not sure the modeling, particularly by the rambunctious and unruly fifth-grade boys (and they are *all boys*), is exactly what I'd hope for, but Ben loves it all. Watching him, I love it all, too.

WEDNESDAY, OCTOBER 10, 2012

I was tucking Ben in just now, and he gave me a *huge* hug and kiss. I grinned ear to ear.

He grinned back and exclaimed, "I love it when you're happy!"

"Awwww," I responded, heart swelling.

"As opposed to when you're mean and grouchy," he concluded.

Yikes!

"I'll work on that," I replied.

"I know you will," he answered.

Sean asked me, "How's it feel to be zinged by your son?"

Heaven. Pure heaven.

SUNDAY, OCTOBER 21, 2012

I was in a three-car collision last week. The car in front of me slowed to allow a propane truck to exit a driveway, so I slowed as well. But the woman behind me was texting and didn't slow down. She smashed into me and pushed me into the car in front of me, injuring my neck and back. An ambulance arrived; I was placed on a stretcher and taken to the hospital.

I have been thanking God every day for the accident. I don't know why it happened, but it happened, and I've decided to be happy about it. I know good will come from it, whatever way it comes. I'm embracing it all. Sean is staying happy, too. We may as well. It sounds too new agey for my tastes, but really, what good will anger or self-pity do?

Life hasn't stopped feeling like I'm on fast-forward since we moved from Boston seven weeks ago. And now a car accident. But it's okay. I will catch up. Sean is worried about me and tired. The children are happy. Ben is struggling with some rigidity, some tantrums, and a fair amount of crying lately. It ebbs and flows. I'll figure it out. Or not.

My T-shirt says: "I'm perfect. You adjust." That's life talking to me today.

Ben and Alina are outside, in the driveway, playing basketball together in the dark. Amazing.

SUNDAY, NOVEMBER 4, 2012

Yesterday was Ben's tenth birthday, and without a doubt, the first day of his second decade was one of the best days of his life. Some of our Waldorf-homeschool friends threw a birthday bonfire for Ben. We are in Boston again, courtesy of Hurricane Sandy and the power outage in Chestnut Ridge. Thanks to Sandy, Ben's birthday was a night of miracles. Essentially, Ben spent the evening playing with a group of friends with whom he spent a lot of time last year. Last year was, in fact, the first year Ben had the capacity for friendship. He cultivated relationships with these children over a period of months, and although it was a brief period, they remain real and meaningful connections for him.

Ben reconnected with these friends and spent his birthday evening running around with a pack of children, playing, laughing, screaming, dueling with glow straws in Day-Glo colors, and feeling, in my observation, more connected and "a part of" than ever in his young life.

Ben's birthday wish last night was to be with his two buddies on his birthday next year. I sat back and tried to accept what was happening and let go of my feelings of waiting for the other shoe to drop. Sean said, "Just enjoy it, honey." I tried.

MONDAY, NOVEMBER 5, 2012

We've been in Boston for over three weeks now, waiting for the power in New York to come back on after the storm. Last night, as I tucked Ben in, I said to him, "I'm so proud of you. You're doing so well, and I mean, you're out of your home, you're out of school, you're out of your routine . . ."

Ben looked at me and said, "And *you're* out of your mind!"

Then he grinned really big. Funny kid.

Then tonight, as I was tucking Ben in and saying prayers, he suddenly interrupted me and said, "Can you stop prayers now? I'm having a meeting with my brain."

Consequences

Ben still hits, bites, and pinches Alina sometimes, and I want him to stop doing that. I have never been disciplined about imposing consequences, but Ben is ready, and it is important. Certain things are off-limits as consequences, because it would cause too much upset, such as taking away foods the kids love, when they have so few choices anyway. But this afternoon, Ben deliberately hit Alina, and I knew something had to be done.

I took away Ben's books for the rest of the day, and right now he is a really sad little critter. Now I have to not cave and let him have his books back. I feel pathetic. The idea of Ben being unhappy for any length of time is harder for me than for him! Not surprising after so many years of autism. But I have to change. I want these kids to be healthy.

SATURDAY, NOVEMBER 10, 2012

Sean and I went out tonight with some new friends from Alina's school. We hired a new babysitter. Ben had never met her before today. She arrived at 4:30, and I explained the evening routine to her. We said goodbye to the kids and left. Three and a half hours later, we returned. *Nothing had happened.* No incidents. The children and the babysitter played and had fun together. The house was tidied up, and things were peaceful.

A year ago, an evening like this would have been iffy.

Two years ago, an evening like this would have been extremely unlikely.

Three, four, five-plus years ago, an evening like this would have been utterly impossible.

Until a few years ago, Ben had crying and screaming fits constantly, sometimes on a daily basis, lasting up to forty minutes at a time.

Until a year or two ago, Ben did not relax and welcome people into our home, and frightened off any babysitters who did not know how to handle a child who did not acknowledge their presence.

But today, Ben, my special-souled ten-year-old, is able to connect, interested in others, and no longer a barrier to a night out with friends for Sean and me.

SUNDAY, NOVEMBER 11, 2012

Tucking Ben in tonight, I said, "Ben, can I have a hug?"

We hugged, and he wouldn't let me go. I stayed and waited.

"Don't ever leave," Ben said. "I want to stay like this until I die!" Seeing my startled eyes, he paused, enjoying the shock value of his own words, a mischievous smile lighting up his face.

"That means," he clarified, "that I love you."

Alina needs love, too. Earlier, during prayers and singing, she watched me stroke Ben's hair, a slight frown on her face. Noticing, I left Ben's side and came to her. I stroked her hair. Her sudden smile could have lit up the post-Sandy Jersey Shore.

SATURDAY, NOVEMBER 24, 2012

We just got back from three days in Rhode Island, where we spent Thanksgiving with Sean's family. It was the first time we have ever spent two nights there. It went off without a hitch.

We held a dinner with ten people for Thanksgiving, and the children behaved beautifully. Ben had no tantrums, he stayed responsive and interactive, and when I took the children to get their hair cut yesterday, they waited patiently while Mommy got a blow-dry. I mentioned to the stylist doing my hair, who had also cut Ben's hair, that Ben used to have autism. Her eyes widened considerably, and she exclaimed, "Well, you've done a *great* job!"

Sean's father, the kids' Zayde, a brilliant attorney and a stickler for realistic thinking (read: he never really thought Ben would recover), was impressed. Ben gave him lots of hugs, and, in one of the best moments ever, Ben threw Zayde a no-delay high-five when Zayde put up his hand as Ben passed in front of him. Later in the day, Grandma Ro exclaimed to us, "That boy just used colloquial language!"

Then when we were leaving this morning, Ben ran over to hug Zayde goodbye and pretended to cry big tears, with his hands in fists on his cheeks. Zayde beamed.

Ben still has huge issues: attention span, rigidity, being unable to locate things (like where the forks are kept in the kitchen even though we have lived here for three months), and emotional upheaval to the point of hysteria if he gets too hungry. But he is making real progress.

I still question whether New York is the right landing pad for us. But until next June, I'm acting as if we are here to stay, and I will see what God shows me in the interim.

TUESDAY, NOVEMBER 27, 2012

Ever since we went to Thanksgiving at Sean's parents' home in Rhode Island, Ben has felt off. He hasn't behaved badly, but he seems off.

His obsession with books has also become problematic. He ignores anyone who tries to interrupt his reading, and lately I have to literally pull the book away before he will acknowledge my existence. Tonight we had quite an exchange. He wanted to read a little more after Alina fell asleep. Sean is away on business this week. I told Ben he could read for five more minutes. I left the room, chatted with Sean on the phone, and came back eight minutes later. I said, "Hey, I gave you three extra minutes. Let's turn out the light." Ben replied, "I only have a little more?" I looked and saw that, indeed, he only had one or two more pages in the book. "Oh, no problem sweetheart," I said. "I'll just wait while you finish."

A moment later, I looked down, and Ben had flipped backwards in the book, so that he now had about seven or eight pages left. "Wait a minute!" I cried. "That is not okay! You said you just had a page or two more!" Ben refused to stop reading, and when I tried to take the book, he clutched it tightly. "Ben," I said, exasperated, "this is unacceptable. You told me you had not much left, now you have made it so you have a lot left. Give me the book!"

We went back and forth a bit, both of us getting more and more rigid (great modeling, I know). Finally, Ben play-punched me in the chest, and I lost it. I grabbed the book, stomped out, went into the kids' bathroom right next door, put the book on the sink, and flushed the toilet. I marched back into Ben's room and announced that I had flushed his book down the toilet. Ben's face crumpled, and he started crying. Big, fat, crocodile tears. Like Alina, however, Ben believes his own performances, so that inevitably, the line between acting and actual emoting blurs. What begins as a snowball at the top of the mountain ends up as an avalanche of hysteria by the time it reaches the bottom.

Sure enough, Ben was absolutely heartbroken. "Did you really flush it down the toilet?" "Yes. I did," I lied. "Then you must want your son to die, and to have no son at all!" "Yes, that is exactly what I want. Give me a break, Ben. You're being as bad as Alina with all this melodrama! You are constantly rude to everybody when you read. I don't know if it's autism, or if you are just being rude, but I think it's just you being rude because when you want to, you just stop reading. People are more important than things, Ben, but you don't act like that!"

Out it gushed, this dreck, filled with truths but inappropriately expressed, and he couldn't hear it anyway, so bereft was he at losing his precious book.

Finally I ran out of steam and said, softly now, "Maybe it is the autism still, BenBen. Maybe it feels really hard to interrupt what you're doing when you're reading. Maybe it's hard for your brain to change gears. I don't know." Ben stared at me.

"I think it's because of Rhode Island," he replied.

"What do you mean?" I asked.

"I think it's not good for me to travel," he responded. I was so touched by his willingness to look at himself and take ownership of his behavior, and by his sheer honesty, that I stopped short and admitted I hadn't flushed the book. It was as if all the orchestras of heaven had begun to play. Wide-eyed, he asked, "Really? You didn't flush it?"

"No, silly," I replied. "How could I flush that big book down a little toilet hole?"

Then I took the opportunity to say, gently and sanely, that people are more important than things, that it's not really fun to do things alone in life compared to having someone to share things with. Ben suddenly burst into laughter. I asked, "Ben, why are you laughing at this? It's not really funny." Ben became serious again and replied, "I don't know. I think it was just a gift of laughter that the angels sent to me, because they saw me so sad before."

Okay.

We are supposed to go to Washington, DC, to my parents' home, for five days next month. We are also planning to go to Florida for four days in February over the children's winter break, to stay with Sean's parents at their condo in Fort Lauderdale. After our rather heated exchange this evening, I asked Ben about both of those trips, and he said he wasn't sure whether he should go on either one. Ben is a wise and consistently accurate gauge of his tolerance levels, and I will honor his choices. I told him we didn't need to think about it tonight, but that we would do whatever felt right, even if it meant his not going. He thanked me, relaxed, and finally settled into bed, ready for sleep.

THURSDAY, NOVEMBER 29, 2012

There is something different in Ben lately. It's hard to put into words. There is a subtle quality to his presence now that signifies a new and greater progress than I have seen before. There is a constant expression of love, for one thing. Tonight, Sean told me that when he went in to kiss Ben good night, he asked Ben how he was feeling. Ben replied, "Good, but I'm cold!" "You are, Ben? Do you want me to turn up the heat?" Sean asked. "No!" Ben exclaimed, and threw his arms wide open in an invitation to a hug, which was the whole point of Ben's saying he was "cold."

Earlier this evening, Ben, Alina, and I sat on the couch reading together, very cozy, and Ben suddenly laughed and blurted out, "Look!" When my eyes followed his finger, which was pointing downward, I saw it was pointing to the word "Susan" there in his book. "You are so sweet!" I exclaimed, hugging him tightly to me.

This afternoon, we had a playdate with the newest, and only other male, member of Ben's class, the wondrous Max, with whom Ben has fallen in a friendship-crush. Toward the end of the afternoon, Max fell off Ben's scooter, which he had been riding, and injured his knee. Apparently, Ben, on the other side of the driveway, didn't notice Max's distress. I can totally imagine this, as Ben still has moments where he is oblivious to the world around him.

I was on the phone inside the house, when suddenly I heard Max screaming and crying. I ran out and saw Max lying prone on our sofa, crying his eyes out. When I ran over, Max yelled out, "Why didn't Ben notice I got hurt? Why didn't he ask me if I was okay? Doesn't he want to be my friend anymore? I think he doesn't want to be my friend anymore!" Stunned by this outpouring of emotion and vulnerability, I knelt down beside him to reassure him that Ben still wanted to be his friend and that I was sure Ben would tell Max as much once he arrived.

Sure enough, Ben soon came running in. He immediately apologized to Max, saying, "I'm sorry I didn't come over right away, Max! I didn't know you had gotten hurt. I was on the other side and didn't see you! I'm sorry!" I said, carefully, "Ben, Max was worried you didn't want to be his friend anymore and that's why you didn't come over." "Yeah," confirmed Max.

Ben moved closer and said, "Of course I still want to be your friend. Nothing could make me not want to be your friend. I care about you, Max."

I nearly fell over.

This school, as much as I don't want to admit it (because I really want to live in Boston and not New York), is *working* for Ben. He's blossoming.

Later, I asked Max if he would want to come back for another playdate even though he got hurt today, and he said he would. Thank God!

I'm powerless. I can't save or fix these kids. I can love them, pray for them, work hard for them, believe in them, and cheer them on no matter what. Only God can heal them. But I am a part of it.

SATURDAY, DECEMBER 8, 2012

I tried giving Ben some new foods this week: apples, raw carrots, and pistachios. All bombed; nonresponsiveness and tantrums came back. I think we are just going to stick with our same old, same old GAPS 1 to 3 Intro Stages. Ben said to me, "It's okay, Mommy. I'm really not tired of the same foods I've been eating." I think he just wants to be able to be present. He ignored me earlier today when I asked him a question, and when I confronted him about it, he commented, "I really don't think I was being rude. I think it was really something causing me a problem."

We had a Hanukkah party this afternoon with Ben's classmates, a friend of Alina's, and lots of parents. It went really well, and Ben and Alina both had a blast. We played *dreidel*, lit candles, and even did a little Hanukkah play. Nice to be able to have a semi-normal family life.

WEDNESDAY, DECEMBER 19, 2012

I finally created a recipe for a cookie that the children can tolerate without a bad reaction ("bad reaction" equals autistic behaviors from Ben and bloating and mood swings for Alina). They love these things, which are made of coconut flour, egg yolks, camel milk, walnuts, and stevia. Two nights ago, I yelled: "It's cookie cleanup! If we can clean the playroom in under five minutes, you guys get cookies!" "*Yay!*" the children yelled, and we hammered the cleanup in less than five minutes.

So then last night, pleased with the previous night's success, I again yelled, "It's cookie cleanup time!" Alina yelled, "Yay!" Ben, on the other hand, became very serious and asserted, fiercely, "No. We cannot do that. We can clean up, but not for cookies. I won't do it for cookies!"

Curious, I followed him into the playroom. "Ben, why don't you want to have a reward for doing a good job cleaning up?" "Because, Mommy," he said patiently, as if to a small and inexperienced child, "we shouldn't clean up for a reward. We should clean up because it's the right thing to do."

In a walk-in closet, I gave birth to Pollyanna.

For my part, I apologized to Ben for my misguided, poorly thought-out attempt to bribe him and his sister to do what he very appropriately said they should do because it's the right thing to do.

Alina was, of course, furious at the whole conversation. That's my girl.

Normal life, sort of

These days we are dealing with the following:

- Sibling rivalry
- She can eat this, but he can't; he can eat that, but she can't
- Daddy's away every other week, and we miss him terribly
- We're all fighting colds and coughs
- Daily enemas that we have to do as part of the CD protocol

Pretty normal stuff. (Except, of course, the enemas.)

FRIDAY, DECEMBER 21, 2012

Alina and I are traveling to Washington, DC tomorrow for a holiday visit and to see The Nutcracker with Grandpa Herman. Sadly, Ben and Sean were to accompany us, but both are too sick to go, especially Sean. Tonight when we were tucking in the children, Ben threw his arms around me and pretended to cry. I said, "I love you, BenBen." He replied in a high, deliberately whining and sad voice, "*I loooooooooooove you toooooooooo and I don't think I can bear being away from you for so long!*"

Hanukkah came early for Mommy.

DECEMBER 2012

Yeast flare-up—I think

Ben has been showing autistic behavior for the past week and a half. He is still fully interactive, expressive, funny, engaged, doing his work, and "with us." A year or two ago, I would have traded an arm for Ben's current level of functioning. But Ben has recovered further, and thankfully, my standards are higher.

Ben has also been fatigued, nonresponsive at times, and extremely distracted. He plays with his shoes instead of paying attention to what is in front of him to be done. At school he wanders off and lies down on the floor. At home he has fits of hysterical laughter. He has also been very aggressive with Alina, pinching and even hitting her (gently but painfully, and enough to make her afraid) on a daily basis.

The nonresponsiveness, hysteria, and distractedness all present like a yeast flare-up. The aggressive fatigue seems due to a bad cold he's had, plus the yeast, which saps his energy by interfering with his immune system and neural functioning.

So now I am a detective again. If I am right, and a major part of this is yeast, what is causing this yeast flare-up?

FRIDAY, DECEMBER 28, 2012

One night last week, I had a sudden epiphany that CD works by oxidizing bad bacteria out of the body, and the walnuts—one of the highest antioxidant-bearing foods—that Ben has been mainlining for the past month were probably interfering with the effect of the CD. So the parasites were most likely in full swing again.

Oops?

I spoke to Sean, and we immediately took both children off the walnuts. Alina's bloat diminished a bit, and Ben almost immediately—within a day or two, that is—"returned" to us, back into responsiveness, eye contact, and connection.

But now, for the past two to three days, Ben has again been rigid, short-fused, throwing tantrums, and even physically aggressive with Alina, pinching and pushing her, though never to the point of injury. But it's startling. Ben's typically gentle, even fragile at times, but right now he is like an addict in withdrawal, downright mean sometimes, and upsetting to see him behave this way. I think he is experiencing withdrawals from the walnuts.

I keep hoping for the day when I can give the children a wider diet. At this point, however, I need to stay put and do what I know will help, not harm. It's so hard sometimes! I want to give them "normal" stuff. But we have to wait.

Patience, I am praying for you in this fast-approaching new year. Patience to find a home. Patience for Sean to possibly find a new job, if that is what we decide is right for all of us. Patience for my body to heal and grow strong again after the car accident. Patience for the children to get what they need medically, physically, emotionally, and educationally. Patience for Ben to fully recover from autism. Patience to embrace, with joy and appreciation, everything exactly as it is and as we are, right now.

MONDAY, DECEMBER 31, 2012

Sean asked at dinner that we each share three things for which we were grateful from the year 2012. Alina's comments were focused largely on the rest of us. I said I was grateful for the move to New York, homeschooling the children last winter, and the happy times this year with Sean. Sean said he was grateful for how well the children have adapted to New York, for the biomedical treatments we are using, and for his company's support in letting him telecommute.

Ben said, "I am grateful for my adorable little sister, for my parents, and for my birthday party in November with old friends."

Again, the awe. "With old friends." Ben was, of course, referring to his Boston friends, who took us in and feted Ben on his birthday when we were marooned in Boston because of Hurricane Sandy. It was beautiful to hear Ben remember and cherish the memory.

Do families who have not experienced autism appreciate the beauty and poignancy of children and their emotions, their love, and what they share with us?

SUNDAY, JANUARY 6, 2013

I am tired.

I am tired of this journey. Not of parenting, or marriage, or life and spiritual growth.

I am tired of the exhaustion that comes with trying too hard, not giving things time to gel, to foment, to slowly, organically, and gently unfold. I need to have the slogan "Time takes time" tattooed on my arms. I don't wait for things to happen in their own time. I rush, push, and complicate. I introduce new ideas, directions, and approaches, and I lose clarity.

I need more faith. I need more trust.

TUESDAY, JANUARY 8, 2013

Ben has been laughing manically for two days straight. Last night he didn't fall asleep until close to 10:30 because he couldn't stop laughing. Now it's almost 9, and he can't stop.

Bizarre to the uninitiated. To us? It's just yeast.

I feel jaded. Where have the wonder, awe, and confusion gone? Too much time spent watching, observing, studying, and scrutinizing the behavior and interactions of my beloved son.

I'm sick of it!

I am considering returning to SCD and dumping GAPS. Ben can't eat many of the GAPS foods anyway, and there is something new now called "Enhanced SCD," which is supposedly helping many children with autism.

Here we go round the mulberry bush, the mulberry bush, the mulberry bush . . .

SUNDAY, JANUARY 13, 2013

Pancakes, parasites, and PANDAS

Ben's autism has kicked up again. Circuiting (running manically back and forth through the house, in circles, laughing, pensive, remote, and driven); auditory-response delays; spacey-ness; periods of extreme rigidity; and most eerie, a blast from the past, two straight days of nonstop giddy and uncontrollable laughter—up all night laughing and unable to stop.

Why is Ben so impaired right now? There are a lot of possibilities, including some anti-parasite medicine a new doctor recently prescribed for Ben. Being on this journey, one of my biggest challenges is frustration at the absolute uncertainty of Ben's progress. One day he seems better and then boom! We are back to autism. We try this intervention and then that one, hoping for the best, and try to stay open and positive.

You might think I'd rather be watching movies, kissing my husband who's away in Boston this week, spending money on "fun stuff" (*e.g.*, clothing, vacations, dinners at fancy restaurants, college funds), and living a different type of life. You might think I was resentful at life because my days and evenings and sometimes even nights are spent reading and researching and talking to people about autism, parasites, and autoimmune disorders, instead of relaxing, kicking back, and letting go. You might think I was filled with self-pity.

You'd be right.

But greater than my resentment or self-pity will ever be is my appreciation for the beautiful people in my life, especially my husband, my children, and my parents. Every evening when I sit and read to the children, I am happy. When Sean and I connect and celebrate each other or apologize for the eightieth cross word or even when I hear his voice on the phone—I'm happy. Love is the goal, and I've got it.

MONDAY, JANUARY 14, 2013

Ben was notably less autistic and less aggressive today. He also did less circuiting. I am mystified.

Maybe he's adjusted to the new homeopathic remedies. Maybe the new parasite medications, which we started last night, are helping. Maybe getting off walnuts, coconut flour, and whatever other foods I am too tired to remember right now is helping. I am trying to enjoy my son in whatever state of mind he happens to be, at whatever moment. I am trying not to wait for someday when he will be "cured" before I love, accept, and join him.

I'm completely confused.

TUESDAY, JANUARY 29, 2013

Tucking Ben in tonight, I remarked to Ben that his intense devotion to Alina reminds me a lot of how my older brother, Danny, felt about me. When we were teenagers, Danny told a neighbor that he wanted to have six children. They all had to be girls, he said, and they all had to be just like me. As I reminded Ben of this story, which he has heard before, Ben's face screwed up into sadness. Danny died after a failed heart surgery when he was sixteen and I was thirteen, and Ben finds the subject of my late brother terribly sad. I tried to explain to Ben, as I often have in the past, that Danny is not a sad presence in my life but a source of happy memories. I had thirteen years with a beautiful person, and some people never get to have a sibling.

As usual, however, Ben wouldn't or couldn't look at Danny from a happy perspective. He started crying, big drops that seemed so exaggerated that they must be crocodile tears but somehow were not. Something about people dying is abjectly heartbreaking to Ben. I don't know why. He said, "If I were you or Grandma Mary or Grandpa Herman, I would kill myself so I could be with Danny!"

Um . . . okay?

"Well, Ben," I attempted further, "Danny lives in my heart, and he was here for the time he was meant to be here. He was meant to be here for sixteen years, and that was his journey."

At this point, Ben went off on this tangent that I tried to understand but really couldn't grasp. He said, "So Danny had a different reason for being here than we do. You and me and Alina and Daddy, we're here to be happy together, to make each other happy. But Danny was here to find his wisdom."

I asked Ben to explain. I told him I understood what he meant about him, Alina, Daddy, and me, but couldn't quite understand what he meant about Danny "finding his wisdom." Ben repeated, "He just was here to find his wisdom. He had a different reason." I still couldn't get it. I reiterated that Danny and I were very happy together, for the time we had one another. But it didn't matter to Ben. He just couldn't take it in.

I wonder what Ben meant by 'Danny's purpose was to find his wisdom.' His consistently inconsolable sadness—almost as if he had known Danny and lost him himself—upon any mention of Danny is both puzzling and moving. He has such empathy, but why choose such a sad outlook?

The intensity of Ben's feelings seems overwhelming to him, and I don't like the idea of such extreme emotion taking him over in that way. Ben's emotional response seemed, as I noted above, almost fake, it was so strong. But he really feels it. Autism? Immaturity? Childhood? Fear of his own mortality or the thought of losing his own close family members?

Whatever it is, he is certainly not emotionally remote anymore!

THURSDAY, JANUARY 31, 2013

Per our DAN! doctor's suggestion, we are attempting to cut out potential problem-causing elements in Ben's current treatment protocol to assess what has triggered his massive deterioration in gut ecology, which has been accompanied by a return to many autistic symptoms we have not seen in literally years.

Once we get Ben back to a gut-healthy state, I will assess the best healing diet for him. I believe GAPS is healing, but somehow the chemistry has not worked for Ben thus far, and the rigidity of his nutrient intake is greatly troubling. So I don't know what to do diet-wise, but once he's healthier, we'll assess.

FRIDAY, FEBRUARY 1, 2013

This morning Ben had a complete autistic fit when he couldn't remember the name of one of the characters (a cat) in a story from yesterday. He repeatedly screamed, "What's the cat's name?! What's the cat's name?!" Over and over again. Then he demanded of Alina, "What's the cat's name, Alina? Alina, what's the cat's name, Alina?" (Ben often says the name of the person to whom he's speaking at both the beginning and the end of his sentences.) Alina responded that she had no idea, and Ben grabbed her and tried to shake it out of her. I told Alina to go to her room and shut the door, because Ben was having a problem. She ran away, upset by Ben's attack.

Seeing Ben so out of control, I panicked. I grabbed Ben and forcefully put him into his bedroom, where I yelled, "*You cannot touch your sister like that! You may not do that! I am taking you out of school and putting you back into Son-Rise!*"

Ben looked horrified, probably more by my behavior than my words. I left the room, upset at both of us and the situation. Ben came out, and I squatted down to be on his level, took him gently by his shoulders, and explained, "Ben, I'm so sorry I lost my temper." Ben, with the saddest expression on his face, replied, "I'm so sorry I lost *my* temper. I don't know why I am doing these things. What's wrong with me?" I replied that we are seeing a lot of autism now because we are missing something. Something is not working, and I have not figured it out yet, but I would. Ben commented, "It must be the food!" I said maybe, but that we would figure it out, and that was a promise.

We were stable for the rest of the morning. Alina recovered, and we got to school on time.

FRIDAY, FEBRUARY 1, 2013

Ben is on heavy-duty parasitic medications from a new doctor, and I think they are too strong for his system and are triggering autistic symptoms in him.

SATURDAY, FEBRUARY 2, 2013

Ben seemed a tiny bit better today, though he has been hit with a huge, whopping cold, complete with headache, congestion, and overall misery. He is blowing his nose so much that his nostrils are flaming red, and the middle section of his nose is white. Poor baby.

This morning as I left for a meeting, I called out, "I love you guys!" and Ben replied, quietly, with a sweet look on his face, "I love you, too, Mommy." It startled me a little; he's been so consumed with nonstop storytelling that I did not expect any response whatsoever to my farewell, much less an expression of love.

I cried with frustration today. I have a stomach flu, and I think it made me emotional. At one point I was in a lot of pain and had to interrupt a story-telling session with Ben. I told him I needed to use the bathroom because my stomach hurt so much. He just ignored me, as if I hadn't said anything, and continued the story. I said, "Ben, didn't you hear me? I'm in pain! Don't you care that I'm in pain?" Ben just continued the story with no break.

SUNDAY, FEBRUARY 3, 2013

Today Ben was slammed again with the virus: fever, huge congestion, and total exhaustion.

I recently learned how the massive amounts of meat children consume on SCD and GAPS can be harmfully acidifying, and am heading toward the Body Ecology Diet to alkalize Ben's gut. An overly acidic gut is a breeding ground for unhealthy bacteria, such as yeast. I told Ben on Body Ecology, we need to do 80 percent vegetables and 20 percent meat, which means trying more vegetables. He was open to it.

MONDAY, FEBRUARY 4, 2013

Ben is still sick. Overnight very high fever, which broke this morning. All day long horrendous congestion with a nose so raw it was painful for me to look at. Thank God he knows how to blow his nose.

TUESDAY, FEBRUARY 5, 2013

Ben and I are still sick with our respective viruses. Today he was much better but completely in rigid-game mode. In other words, he wanted me, he was not exclusive at all, but he was and is utterly, utterly obsessed with story telling about Bobby, A.M., and another line of stories based on Daisy Meadows's fairy-story chapter books. I was completely in Ben's world all day long. There is no playroom—the entire house is Ben's playroom now, and I am his Son-Rise Program facilitator from 7 AM until he drops off around 7:30 PM. We are having endless fun with the variations on the stories. In the early years of our Son-Rise Program, I would have had a harder time, but I am relaxed now, so it's actually fun.

Alina told Sean and me tonight as we were tucking her in that she is sick of hearing us talk about Ben this, Ben that, and so forth. We reassured her that we love her too, and I celebrated her for speaking up and telling us how she feels. We work very hard to let her know we cherish her, and she is, thank God, a happy child. She even overcame a situation at school with a little boy who was bullying her, and they are now pals!

TUESDAY, FEBRUARY 5, 2013

Two nights ago, when Ben was terribly sick with fever, I tucked him in next to me, said prayers, and sang a little bit. Then I said, "Good night, BenBen." Ben replied, "Good night, Mommy."

Ben replied, "Good night, Mommy."

It was the most natural, beautiful, and innocent expression of love I have ever heard. In his little-boy voice, my son said, "Good night, Mommy."

I know non-ASD parents don't empathize with my heartbreak and heart healing in the way ASD parents do, but any parent on earth understands the force of receiving love from your child. I lay in bed, replaying his words, his tone, and his connection with me, over and over in my mind until I, too, fell asleep.

Ben's fever broke the next morning.

WEDNESDAY, FEBRUARY 6, 2013

Alina is soaring in every area in school except for her physical fitness, specifically agility and cardiovascular capacity. She has a metabolism that seems to be completely stalled out, and although she eats nothing that is not healthy, and in not very substantial amounts, she continues to gain weight and be bloated. So movement is harder for her than if she were healthy. We continue to explore avenues of healing for Alina as well as Ben.

We did a few more baby carrots today (cooked). We added sunflower butter (I found some that has no sugar), which he loved. It's relatively alkalizing, so I'm pleased to use it instead of tahini, which is more acidifying and therefore a poor choice for Ben. Ben also ate cooked cauliflower with flax oil and salt and tried an apricot-flaxseed bar, which he *loved*. We'll see if there is a reaction, but it was a blast to see him light up with joy when he (1) saw the bar (wrapped up and looking like a regular kid's store-bought snack) and (2) ate the thing and loved it. He circuited a bit less today, was responsive at times and not there at other times, but overall, was in a better space.

That's enough. I'm tired and going to watch *Downton Abbey*.

THURSDAY, FEBRUARY 7, 2013

Coloring books and serial killers

Ben was able to do half a day of school today. He designed a math quiz for his classmates that showcased things each of them loves, in each of the respective math problems. Each equation read something like this:

For Tanya, who loves coloring books:

"If you have 24 coloring books, and you add four more, how many coloring books do you have?"

For Anjana, who loves Shetland ponies:

"If you have 15 Shetland ponies, and you get 10 more, how many Shetland ponies do you have?"

The funniest of all were the equations Ben wrote for his friend, Max, who loves anything to do with blood and gore. It read as follows: "If you have 27 serial killers, and you get 14 more, how many serial killers do you have?"

He typed it all up on my laptop yesterday afternoon, printed out five copies, and brought them in for everyone to read. He articulately and clearly explained what the exercise was, and the children all enjoyed it very much.

It's so ironic: Ben designed a theme! He took each of his friends, identified their motivators, and got them to work on a difficult skill (math) by incorporating their respective motivators into the exercise.

I'm so proud of my junior Son-Rise Program facilitator!

THURSDAY, FEBRUARY 7, 2013

Today I took time off for me and didn't pay attention to Ben much at all. I felt guilty, but it was a good day. I promised him tomorrow I will be more present and available. I have decided to completely discontinue the heavy-duty anti-parasitics, which seem to be way too intense for Ben. I also didn't realize that "systemic" means that they get into the bloodstream and cross the blood-brain barrier. Not a good choice for Ben, who is still so delicate. Also, x-rays on the children's respective digestive tracts have revealed large fecal blockages (read: old poop), which have to be removed with hydrotherapy. I expect I will be doing it, too.

Some families go to Disney.

FRIDAY, FEBRUARY 8, 2013

Today we got pummeled by Snowstorm Nemo, which is slamming the East Coast. Mom and Dad are treating us to a hotel, to avoid power-outage misery. Sean and Alina are in Florida.

Right now Ben is very autistic. He doesn't notice when other people are talking; he interrupts and is totally unaware he is interrupting. I allowed Ben an hour of computer time today, mostly because I fell asleep. He circuited intensely, with a focused and intense look on his face as he did. Yet he was very affectionate and at times talked with me about topics having nothing to do with his stories. Confusing.

SATURDAY, FEBRUARY 9, 2013

I spent today joining with Ben in his rigid game. From 9 AM until 7:30 PM, we told stories about Bobby, A.M., and Fluffer. This particular storyline is always the same joke: Bobby Mall, a mean-spirited older brother, delights in torturing his younger sister, A.M. (short for Ally Mall). A.M. is a member of Ms. Pearl's class, whose class pet is

Fluffer, the runt of a litter of eleven male snowy-hound puppies. Every weekend, one of Ms. Pearl's 100 first-grade students (it's a big class . . .) has the privilege of taking Fluffer home. Fluffer also goes home with a student on holiday breaks. Every time it is A.M.'s turn to bring Fluffer home (the opening to every story Ben tells), Bobby is furious, as are his eleven "mutts," who are as mean-spirited as their master, Bobby, and taunt Fluffer endlessly.

A.M. also has a best friend named John, who is in another class, taught by Ms. Pourin. John and A.M. are allies against Bobby and John's older sister, Sarah, who is Bobby's girlfriend. Bobby and Sarah are students at "Knighting School," which is held on Saturn (the planet). Whenever things are not to their liking at home, Bobby and Sarah fly off to Knighting School in a rocket ship. At Knighting School, the children eat hot dogs, French fries, chocolate bars, and drink Coca-Cola. They study fighting, and Bobby's mutts are welcome. Fluffer is not. The story is informed by my joke telling, which frequently sends Ben into fits of spasmodic laughter, often ending up in total hysteria. It's pretty fun. Almost always, Ben seizes on one particular (stupid) joke I insert into the story and that becomes our main theme.

Ben told Sean, who is stranded until Monday evening with Alina in Florida because of the blizzard, that today was one of the best days of his life because of our Son-Rise Program time, which was the entire day. I know how he feels when I show up for him this way, when I don't distract myself by other items on my to-do list, and when he is my top priority.

At about 5:30, however, I hit a wall. I wanted to cry. I was sick of story telling and of repeating the same exact jokes for the sixth day in a row (Ben got sick last Monday, was out of school the whole week, and I was his Son-Rise Program the whole time). I told him I needed a break, and he went into the other room to read.

I made dinner, and after getting some calories in me, I was ready for more stories. We did more together, now involving dancing around the room (Bobby/Sarah and A.M./John each had new dances they were using to bother the other pair, respectively), for the next hour or so, until it was time for Ben to go to bed.

From a Son-Rise Program perspective, it was a great day. Ben was more responsive than he's been for a while. But he is still very autistic. Circuiting, general nonresponsiveness, uncontrollable laughter, eyes going all over the ceiling at times, and a certain rigidity and irritability all let me know he is not in a good place. So we have our plan. We know what we're doing for the next two months. I don't know *what* to do about his food; on that point I am extremely confused. I felt a little self-pitying and a bit despondent, but mostly just exhausted this evening. A talk with Sean restored my hope. We have a plan.

Notably, Ben chose to speak with Grandma Mary on the telephone and was more engaged than he has been with any of the grandparents in weeks.

SUNDAY, FEBRUARY 10, 2013

Today was another day of nonstop story telling with Ben. I was so tired that I had to pause at certain points during the day and take a breather, because I had no reserves left.

My mind is spinning with a few thoughts. Acceptance of Ben means loving him now and enjoying our time together without judging him or his autism. But my ability to accept and love also feels contingent on my faith that he can get better. Does that mean my love is conditional, or does it instead mean that my faith must precede my love, otherwise my fear takes over and there is no room for love?

We were driving today to a toy store, and I said to Ben, "I have loved this time alone with you, just you and me, Ben. It has been so special." Ben replied, "To me too." I continued, "It means so much to me to be with you like this." Ben further responded, "You mean a lot to me too, Mommy."

The Son-Rise Program is powerful, and I never understood before how to just be and love in the playroom. Now after seven straight days of nonstop, all-day playroom time, I get it. There's love and there's play, and they come together and that's what heals these children. Heals *my* child. And I'm allowed to take breaks. I bet he's amazing at school tomorrow. He was utterly transformed on the phone tonight with Sean and Alina, talking a blue streak, teasing, and appropriately playful.

MONDAY, FEBRUARY 11, 2013

Today Ben was palpably better, though still showing a lot of autism. He was nonresponsive, didn't answer when I asked him a question, and interrupted conversations with verbal isms as if no one had been talking. *But* . . . he was much more present, flexible, interactive, and the eye contact was consistent and unsolicited. Off the medications, he is definitely coming back to us. Tonight I wished him sweet dreams and told him again what a joy it has been to have this time together, and he replied, "Sweet dreams to *you*, Mommy!"

This morning he made a valentine for his teacher: "Thank you for teaching us. Going to school is the best present I could ever get."

FRIDAY, FEBRUARY 15, 2013

Yesterday was Valentine's Day. Ben made a valentine for each of his classmates, specifically tailored to each person:

(1) To Tori:

Dear Tori, When I first met you I found you to be mean, bullying, and an enemy. But a weekend and a week after Max arrived, you became a good friend. Actually you are now my best friend. I hope we are in the same class next year. Happy Valentine's Day. Love, Ben.

(2)   To Max:

Dear Max, At first we were friends, but then angriness came. I hope we can go back to being friends. Happy V.D. Like, Ben.

(3)   To Tanya:

Dear Tanya, Happy Valentine's Day. I bet this is the day your parents and big brother love you the most. Keep smiling. Love, Ben.

(4)   To Anjana:

Dear Angena, Happy Valentine's Day. Say hi to Cranberry and Lulu for me. Smiles from my heart, Ben.

SATURDAY, FEBRUARY 16, 2013

I have no idea how Ben is doing right now. One minute he's circuiting, in his own world, nonresponsive, and autistic. Next minute he's interactive, engaged, clever in his discourse, and very "with it." Not seeming autistic. Sean and I are baffled. *There are too many factors to consider!* Today, at times, I felt like I was losing it. I am harsh with Alina because I feel so powerless over Ben that I want to exert power *somewhere*. It's terrible, and thankfully I realized what I was doing and stopped treating her badly. But she is smart and perceptive, and I don't want her feeling shaky about our relationship.

I am short-tempered, irritable, and hurting. I want him to be all better. It's already been such a long journey, with so much progress and hope, and then we crash. I am aware I have lost perspective. It's possible I just need some time away to regroup. I have also fallen into an old behavior of over-committing myself, which leaves me no room to feel, no room to breathe, and no way to enjoy my life. I have to accept once again that my life still needs to be focused on Ben's recovery.

MONDAY, FEBRUARY 18, 2013

I feel constantly guilty for playing with Alina, while Ben is doing autism in the background. As if Ben's needs were the only ones, because Alina is not autistic. It's terribly difficult; I feel my duty toward Ben, but obviously Alina has needs as well. It is hard to keep perspective when you feel one of your children slipping away from you.

Ben seems to need an all-day Son-Rise Program right now to carry him through the post-meds detox. But he is in school and ecstatic to be so, and that's where he belongs and where he wants to be. This is school vacation week, and I have both children, as well as an au pair with good intentions but no training yet. So we are all together, and I feel pulled apart: Ben wants story, story, story, and Alina wants me to play Monopoly, dolls, and read out loud to her. I want to be there for Ben and also for Alina. And I love both, and all of it, but I can't be two people at one time. Today, in a fit of impatience to have my attention, Ben screamed out, "Just *clone yourself!!!*"

Then, too, I have my twelve-step program commitments, physical therapy and acupuncture for my back three to five days a week since the car accident, and a marriage, social life, and school commitments to meet. Then it gets to be 9 at night, and I'm so darn tired, and I just want to relax and unwind with television, but it's too late and I have a headache. And I need to write, to document Ben's status and my mental health. And now it's almost ten o'clock and I am shot, and that alarm is going off only too soon.

Despite my complaining, there's no place I'd rather be. I try to find God in my life. I need to back off *more*. Stop thinking I'm driving the car for these children. There's a difference between showing up with love and pushing, pushing, and pushing. It's so hard for me to let go sometimes. Sean sees progress in Ben since last week, and I think he's right. Sean said he remains hopeful and optimistic.

I'm going away next week for five days to see some friends, take a break, and get some sleep.

TUESDAY, FEBRUARY 19, 2013

Ben's behavior today was erratic. One minute he was connected and affectionate. Then he had sudden fits of frustration and rage with Alina. He was intensely rigid at times, then melting away into flexibility and finding solutions where there were none. He was back and forth, in and out of autistic rigidity and amazing flexibility. At nighttime, I told Ben I was sorry I have been spending more time with Alina than with him, and he replied, "It's okay, Mommy. I understand."

Tomorrow Alina and I are going to the American Girl Doll store in Manhattan. I'm nervous and excited.

WEDNESDAY, FEBRUARY 20, 2013

A week ago Ben clearly stated he had no interest in going with us to the American Girl Doll store in the city. Then yesterday, he changed his mind and decided to come. When I asked Alina if she minded Ben going with us, as it was supposed to be our special day together, she replied, "I would love for him to come, Mommy. I wanted him to come from the start." Happy me, to have children who love each other.

Then we missed the bus to the city. Neither child got upset or frustrated, for which I celebrated them royally. "You guys are awesome for being so patient. Thank you!" "Well, I'm feeling a little frustrated, Mommy," Alina confirmed, "but I'm choosing to stay cheerful." Ben just stayed upbeat, period.

Then I, in the words of a dear friend of mine, put on my "big-girl panties" and drove into Manhattan for the first time in my life. It took only forty minutes, we easily found a nearby parking lot, and off down Fifth Avenue we strode, jubilantly arriving at the AGD store less than an hour after we departed from our home. We spent a delighted two hours at the store; Alina got her birthday present—a "Just Like Me" doll whom she named "Alana" ("so we don't get ourselves confused," she explained), who has, like Alina, brown hair, blue eyes, and freckles.

Then, walking back to the parking lot in the freezing cold, Ben and Alina decided to sing the song Ben wrote last week about hugs and tugs of war, in the voices of the Bobby and A.M. characters from Ben's stories. Not only did they sing the song, they actually belted it out all the way down Fifth Avenue, from 49th to 55th. There we were—the children, our au pair, and I—parading down Fifth Avenue, the four of us holding hands, and the children singing this absolutely nutty song at the top of their lungs, while onlookers smiled and grinned at the joy bursting from these children. I was walking on air.

Then, a quick forty-minute ride home, and for the rest of the day the children and I played with Alina's old and new American Girl Dolls. To make it fun for myself—always key when I play with the children—I gave each of the dolls its own distinct personality. Soon the children and I were roaring with laughter. McKenna, my favorite, was flipping her hair over and over again and bossing all of the other dolls around. This sent Ben and Alina into hysterics, as the other dolls criticized McKenna for being so bossy and rude. It's all about hyperbole with my kids (all kids?), and I'm definitely the queen of hyperbole—ask my husband!

Then dinner, cleanup, and bed: an utterly surprising and joy-filled day.

Later we had dinner and, at the end of the evening, read Harry Potter together. Reading Harry Potter represents a major shift for Ben, who has been unwilling to read Harry Potter up until two nights ago, when he decided to give it a try through a negotiation with me to stay up later than I wanted him to that night. Moreover, Ben acknowledged to me that evening that he thought the book would be scary and that was why he didn't want to read it. But he was willing to give it a try!

The first night we read a chapter, Ben inserted Bobby and A.M. language on every page, seemingly per his need to control and dilute the experience of reading this book he thought might scare him. By the second night of reading, however, it was Alina rather than Ben who was inserting the Bobby and A.M. motif, and Ben who sat quietly, in rapt attention, hanging on to every word. I used Ben's apparent interest in the book to do some reading-comprehension work, quizzing the children every few pages about facts I had just read. At the beginning, Ben often missed key pieces, but the more we read, the more Ben's comprehension improved.

Additionally, in the past, Ben has been unwilling to allow people to use accents or funny voices in games or in reading aloud to him. He used to order, on a regular basis, "Use your *regular* voice!" But listening to me read Harry Potter for the past few nights, Ben has not balked at all when I have put on a (truly awful) Scottish brogue for Hagrid and Professor McGonagall and an irritating whine for Dudley Dursley. Ben even commented tonight that A.M. thinks Harry Potter might be better than Rainbow Magic stories. Since A.M. is the voice of goodness and reason in Ben's imaginary world, this constituted high praise.

Then, in a final gesture of flexibility for the evening, Ben agreed to Alina's request to sleep in his room with him tonight, in his trundle bed. He has not been willing to have Alina in his room overnight for a long time.

I am so grateful to see so many gains this week. CD seems to be working again for Ben.

Choosing happiness. Regardless.

Sean cautions me constantly to choose happiness regardless of Ben's daily degree of recovery, but it's hard. I'm too focused on him, and I don't know how to get beyond it, other than through prayer and patience with myself.

FRIDAY, FEBRUARY 22, 2013

Ben loves torturing Alina by telling her how beautiful and lovely and adorable she is, and by endlessly calling her "darling" and "sweetheart" in a sugary-sweet voice. Like all big brothers, he loves driving his little sister crazy!

SATURDAY, FEBRUARY 23, 2013

On our way into Manhattan to go to the American Girl Doll store on Wednesday, the children and I discussed our experience thus far in New York, since the move last September. Ben commented that he prefers New York overall, because it's so fun. "But," he continued, "I had a lot more friends in Boston. I don't have any friends here." My heart stopped. "Well," he continued, "I have a lot of grown-up friends. But I'm not friends with kids."

I was upset to hear Ben saying that he feels he has no friends here in our new home. On the other hand, I was thrilled to hear how much he wants friends. I told him that there was a temple we were considering joining, not too far away in a town called Nyack, where he could go to Sunday school and meet some kids—boys, hopefully— who would be his age. "Would you want to try that, Ben?" I asked. "Yes," he answered. "I would."

Then today, we were talking about our dreams. Alina shared two dreams she has. First, to visit Candyland. Second, to be someone who helps children. Ben said that his dream was to have friends—no shocks there. I will do everything I can to help make that happen. Chess clubs, Hebrew school, playdates—whatever it takes.

SUNDAY, MARCH 24, 2013

One month later

I have not written in a month and a day. I'm burned out, tired, sick of new diets and all of the challenges. I'm watching *Homeland* every night to escape it all.

We have been through so much in 2013 already, with two weeks of anxiety, aggression, and tantrums, and then two weeks of total autism—nonresponsiveness, low eye contact, and utter lack of interest in us. Then, after realizing the error of using systemic anti-parasitics and getting him off those toxic chemicals, two weeks of re-emergence.

Rough start to 2013, but I learned a lot. I saw my own anxiety, aggression, and tantrums. Then I saw my own pseudo-autism: checking out, escaping into television, and isolating into sadness and worry. I am not a perfect spiritual being; I didn't "do it right." But I, too, re-emerged a week or so ago, by opening up to friends again about my fears, my anger, and my dreams.

New diet

Last month, we learned that Ben has an acid Ph in his gut (read: a great, big invitation to toxicity and parasites, and a difficult time colonizing healthy gut flora). Both the Specific Carbohydrate Diet and the GAPS Diet, the two diets we have used over the past five years, are heavily dominated by animal protein. Animal protein creates an acidic blood pH when not balanced by sufficient amounts of alkaline foods, such as fruits and vegetables. Ben has been eating literally pounds of animal-based protein for years. No wonder his gut is so acidic, and no wonder he has such a low nutrient-absorption rate. So I have decided to explore the Body Ecology Diet, which implements primarily alkaline foods. I think we are finally going in the right direction.

How many times have I heard myself saying that exact phrase, "in the right direction"? Or "on the right path"? I guess it doesn't matter. If I didn't have the courage to keep going, exploring, learning, and stumbling forward, Ben might never have come this far.

Miracles do happen. One month and a day ago, Ben told me he wants friends, really badly, and would I please do something about it. So I prayed. The day after that conversation, a new friend here in New York told me about a new program his temple is developing, which he is actually spearheading, to support children with special needs. I met with the rabbi and the educational director the following week to discuss membership at the temple and Ben's involvement in their new program. The following Sunday, Ben joined the temple Sunday school class, where he will now have the opportunity to meet new children and develop friendships.

Tomorrow Ben has a playdate with a new friend, whom I have not met yet but with whom Ben has had a few classes. This Thursday, Ben has a playdate with two new friends, a boy and a girl who have committed to doing playdates every other Thursday with Ben. Prayer works.

Ben is still yeasty, circuiting a little, manic with laughter a lot, and prone to super-intense emotions. Tonight he became inconsolable when I mentioned that he, Ben, loves Alina the way my older brother, Danny, loved me. Ben paused for a minute or so, thinking, and I saw the tide of emotions rising in him. Suddenly, he plunged into a torrent of rather interesting ideas he had about Danny and our family's loss:

First: "How can you be happy?"

Then: "I know this sounds harsh, but maybe I can grow up, have a baby, kill myself, and then Grandma and Grandpa can adopt my child and have a child of their own again!"

Finally: "I want to find an older orphan for Grandma and Grandpa to adopt."

He's like a poster child for an anti-autistic person, my hyper-compassionate, hyper-empathetic son.

SATURDAY, MARCH 2, 2013

I got back from California tonight. The moment I walked through the front door, Ben ran down the hall, calling out, "Mommmmmmmy!" and practically jumped into my arms, covering me with kisses and grinning from ear to ear.

Then at nigh-nighs, he yelled out, "I love you, Mommy!"

Wow!

MONDAY, MARCH 25, 2013

Ben had a playdate with a boy named Kai today, and it went great. They played basketball, then hockey, and then they just hung out in Ben's playroom for a while. Later they helped me make coconut flour cookies for Passover, and Kai loved the cookies! It went really well.

Ben started getting a bit tense toward the end of the afternoon, when Alina, happy in her own playdate with a friend from her second-grade class, came into Ben's playroom. Ben gets a tight, controlling, almost-angry tone at times when he feels threatened. For some reason, I get angry and tight myself when I hear that voice coming out of him. "Darn it, I don't want him to have autism! Don't be so rigid! Don't be so literal and reactive!" Why can't I accept Ben as he is?

Ben had a very big upset today at school. For the first time this year, his teacher called me around 1:30 and suggested I take Ben out of school early. They were discussing the killing of the first-born sons in Egypt, and a girl in Ben's class remarked that it would be great if all the boys were killed. She was just trying to be funny, but Ben took it literally. He got rigid and demanded she change what she had said, and when she wouldn't, he became inconsolable. The teacher said she had never seen Ben unable to let go of something to that degree, and asked could I come pick him up. I responded that I thought Ben should work it through rather than running away. I felt Ben would see it as a failure if I suddenly showed up to take him home. In fact, when I picked him up at the regular time (2:45), he was fine, and the teacher told me he had calmed down after just a little time outside of the classroom.

Where does this rigidity come from? Is he detoxing still? Is it neurological toxicity due to glutathione deficiency? Is it a compromised immune system, or an autoimmune syndrome, PANDAS?

What the hell is it?

WEDNESDAY, MARCH 27, 2013

Tonight we held a Seder with three other families in our new home in New York. Out of fourteen people, five were children. Out of all of the children, Ben was the only one to participate fully and appropriately, reading, singing, and presenting the various parts of the Seder with poise. All the children behaved beautifully. Ben read portions of the Jewish prayer book, joined with great gusto in the holiday songs, and thoroughly enjoyed himself—appropriately. He wasn't too loud, he didn't speak out or interrupt, and he was helpful and kind to everyone.

Now, flash back to Thanksgiving three years ago, which Ben spent underneath the table, while I shuttled plates of food in and Ben pushed them out from underneath the tablecloth. What a difference.

TUESDAY, APRIL 2, 2013

Tonight we started Ben on PharmaNAC, a product that provides L-Acetyl-Cysteine to the body. L-Cysteine is essential to the production of glutathione in the body. Without adequate glutathione levels, the brain cannot detoxify itself sufficiently, and autistic symptoms result. In order for Ben to be willing to take the stuff, which smelled like cherry fizzy water and whose "fizz" was unappealing to Ben, I bribed him with a tiny bit of computer time. To his credit, he only wanted "to do research, not games, Mommy!" He was on my laptop a total of five minutes, and out of it, I earned my right to enforce fizzy water. He drank it unhappily but willingly.

The other part of my bribe reward, however, was even more exciting. Ben does not like to focus in any way on "bad" things. Uncomfortable feelings, hurtful or thoughtless people (unless it's a two-dimensional, caricatured/archetypal, and fictional person either he or another author has created), and any events that he sees as negative are abhorrent to Ben. For example, he refuses to tell Sean or me anything about incidents at school in which he feels he or others have acted poorly. I don't push; I merely call his teacher to get the details.

So today, when I asked Ben how his day at school was, he replied, "A little good." In Ben-speak, that means, "Something bad happened, but I don't want to give you any details." I asked him if anything upsetting had happened, and he confirmed my suspicions by saying, "Yes, but I don't want to tell you about it." I commented, "That's fine, I totally get that. If you change your mind, I'd love to hear what happened. But now let's do a story!" We spent the rest of the afternoon doing stories in the playroom.

Just before dinner, however, Ben got a fierce want to go on the computer and print out some pictures of dogs. He spent the next ten to fifteen minutes trying to get me to let him go on my laptop.

A particularly awesome and hilarious aspect of Ben's negotiation strategy during this ten to fifteen minutes was that while he was trying to get me to cave on the computer issue, he stared right into my eyes, very obviously trying to bribe me with what he knows I constantly want—eye contact! I totally cracked up, telling him, "Oh no, you're not going to get me with your amazing eye contact! Even though it's awesome!"

I was excited. First of all, Ben was aware of my wants. He was also able to fix his eyes on my eyes, nonstop, for a long time, which was not always the case. Best of all, he cleverly attempted to use my wants to get what he wanted!

He was being such a ten-year-old! I loved every minute.

I finally negotiated that if Ben got to go on the computer—definitely a rare event, but I also harbored a fierce want this evening—he would be willing to (1) tell me what had gone wrong today at school, and (2) drink the NAC. Not only that, my demand included him being willing to tell me what happens at school every day—some bad stuff, some good stuff, whatever went down.

After I made my offer, Ben stood, thinking and considering, for a number of moments. I could see the wheels turning in his mind: the struggle between his acute desire for privacy regarding these issues and his intense desire to print out the dog pictures on the computer. Amazingly, Ben agreed to the deal. Not only that, but in typical Ben-fashion, once having let go of having his way, he embraced the new position and suggested that we go to a store before school tomorrow morning to buy a notebook in which he could take notes to report to me about his days after school. I thought the idea was terrific and found him an empty notebook in the house this evening.

Ben finally shared with me about what happened today at school, which arose out of Ben's ongoing super-sensitivity and literality, which are still causing social problems for him. During class this morning,

Ben's teacher made a side comment that all people were wicked at a certain point in time. They were discussing Sodom and Gomorrah in a segment on the Old Testament. But instead of "all people," the teacher said "all men" were wicked. After class, two of the girls in Ben's class were whispering to each other, and Ben listened in. The girls said, "That must be why boys are so annoying!" Ben took the comment personally and assumed the girls were referring to *him* and the other boy in his class. He became upset and demanded that the girls apologize. They had no idea what he was talking about, and the situation escalated.

I commented to Ben that perhaps eavesdropping on the girls' conversations was not helpful and that if he hadn't done so, he wouldn't have heard the comments that were not intended for his ears and that wound up provoking his super-sensitive response. He agreed with me about the listening in and said, "But it's very hard for me not to!" Ben is growing up, interacting with people, and learning as he goes. As are we. It's so cool that he was willing to share what happened at school with me.

FRIDAY, APRIL 5, 2013

I fell off my Son-Rise Program mojo today. Maybe it's the fact that I'm doing a colon cleanse, or the fact that Sean is in Boston and I'm tired, or maybe it's just being the mom of a child I wish didn't have autism. But Ben is Ben, and for today, Ben still has autism.

He lost it today when I let him go on the computer and the pictures he printed—a group of dogs—weren't what he wanted them to be, and I wouldn't let him go back on to print other pictures. Actually, I didn't even refuse his request, but he demanded and yelled that I let him, and I shut down. I got angry. I told him it was unacceptable to speak to me that way, and that he needed to listen to me and not ignore what I was saying. He responded by moaning, through sobs, that he was terrible, evil, and didn't deserve to have me. I told him not to evade what I was saying by going into all that. He paused and considered what I'd said, clearly caught out. He heard me. But it didn't help me; I was just angry.

I felt tired, mad, and disappointed. One minute he's progressing, and the next he's circuiting, rigid, story telling at breakneck pace, needing the story, needing the relief he gets from checking out that way—I just didn't want it to be in him today. I got selfish and thought about what I wanted—instead of loving him.

This evening, while Alina was at a dance class, I asked Ben if we could talk, and he was willing to sit with me on the sofa and have a conversation. I asked him what he thought autism was. He said it's when you can't pay attention. I told him that was right, and that it was also not looking at people and focusing on one thing—getting stuck—so that you can't pay attention to anything else.

I asked him if he saw that in himself. He responded in the affirmative and then gave me an example from today at school, when he got too focused on an idea in his head to pay attention to anything else. He apparently understands what it is to check out, not pay attention, and fixate on one thought. I told him Daddy and I don't see autism as a bad thing; we just don't want him to have it because it takes away some of his choices and might be a problem with friends, girlfriends, and other things he might want to pursue in his life. He seemed to take it in somewhat. But he is still slow to process information like that, and I wonder about my motives in discussing it. Do I want him to get self-aware and therefore be less autistic? Do I want him to make different choices and be less autistic?

Later this evening, I did many stories with him, and he became quite manic. He seems to get manic every evening around 7 to 7:30, just before bedtime. Alina also often does, though Ben's manic stuff involves circuiting madly around the house, story telling in a really loud voice, and laughing crazily. I have gotten angry at the manic behavior sometimes lately, telling him to stop, it's too much, you need to slow down your engine, you sound like a cuckoo bird, Ben, *stop!* Not a lot of patience or tolerance.

Tonight the children started taking their Oxypowder colon-cleanse capsules. It's going to be a fun spring break . . .

SUNDAY, APRIL 7, 2013

Today Ben went and lay down with Sean on the couch to snuggle. Sean melted, his joy palpable. He said to me later, "Ben's never done that before!" Also, today for the second day in a row, Ben was willing to play my new game. The four of us played it last night and today again. Ben acted out Dumbledore, Harry Potter, some characters from his invented world, "Sillian School," and fully participated. It was amazing, the four of us there together, playing a game, having fun, and feeling connected. I felt like a "normal family." Whatever that is.

Then this morning, I was getting dressed. I stood in front of my mirror, putting on some earrings. Ben came into the room, wrapped his arms around me from behind, and said, "You look *great!*" I died. What a moment of happiness. My son thought I looked great. My formerly autistic son *told* me he thought I looked great. Not that we don't still have autism; we do. But to me it's an amalgam of symptoms—not a permanent condition.

There are a lot of moments these days, too many to capture all of them, when Ben's progress is supremely evident. At the same time, his ism, the story telling, is pervasive, nonstop, and desperately needed. I remember my Son-Rise Program teacher telling me that sometimes when there is a big neurological jump forward, there is simultaneously a greater need to ism in order give the brain time to process.

SUNDAY, APRIL 7, 2013

The Body Ecology Diet is having a positive impact. This week, Ben tried snap peas ("I hate to tell you, Mommy, but I don't like my vegetables this sweet!"), Daddy's chicken (ate a bunch for the first time in years), cucumbers (eating them daily now), and is devouring tons of my cauliflower rice (ground up raw, then fried in coconut oil so it looks like rice) every single day, sometimes three times a day. He is eating Go Raw Flax Snax crackers.

I also read this evening that cauliflower, broccoli, walnuts, and avocado all are super foods for boosting glutathione, which is so, so important for Ben. He is currently eating all of those!

MONDAY, APRIL 8, 2013

What is this? It's an empty dish.

Earlier, this evening, this dish was not empty. It was filled with "buckwheat hot cereal," a porridgey-looking stuff, reminiscent of oatmeal and country mornings and that sort of thing. This dish is empty because Ben, my formerly picky eater, ate his whole bowl of stevia-sweetened, buckwheat hot cereal. Never in his life has Ben been willing to eat food of this texture. But tonight he ate it happily. First, he tasted a tiny nibble—barely a bit on the end of his finger. Then, he ate a spoonful. Then, he ate the whole bowl, with gusto. I am starting to believe that anything is possible.

When is an empty dish not just an empty dish? In my home, tonight.

SUNDAY, APRIL 21, 2013

Sean and I agree that Ben seems to have moved forward in his recovery again.

For a few months recently, I felt a certain resignation. Perhaps, I was feeling Ben would get better, but he would remain impaired.

Perhaps he would have a good life, but continue to suffer autistic symptoms that would keep him from becoming a totally fulfilled person, especially socially and interpersonally. Perhaps he would be happy, but limited in his personal and professional possibilities.

Over the last few weeks, however, we have observed subtle-but-meaningful changes. Things that before would have sent him into tantrums or extreme emotions, didn't. When we read, for example, in book three of Harry Potter, that Hagrid's beloved hippogrif, Buckbeak, was executed, Ben didn't get upset. When we have to change gears lately, Ben flows more. When I don't want to do a story with him, he doesn't push back very hard, if at all. He lets go.

At our temple, Ben is showing up enthusiastically and appropriately. Today the Hebrew teacher there said to Sean, "Maybe he'll be the first autistic rabbi!" Sean commented to me that by that point, we hope he will no longer be autistic. I replied, "Perhaps he will be the first *formerly* autistic rabbi!"

He is building new skills. He is at soccer every Saturday, easily the least-skilled player on the field but cheering happily when his team scores a goal and telling other children how well they are doing. He told one girl, who is slightly larger than the other children but gives her heart on the field, that she was "clearly the best player out there today!" The girl grinned brightly in response.

He has a remarkable depth of kindness. Maybe he *will* be a rabbi!

Ben's picky eating seems to be dramatically disappearing. He is willing to taste new foods, repeatedly, and not just a microscopic bit on the tip of his finger. He takes a real bite, is willing to consider the new food for a moment, and responds either positively or negatively, but not unthinkingly, as in the past. He is now eating amaranth (not thrilled), millet (loves it), cucumbers, raw zucchini, red and yellow peppers, cauliflower "rice" (eating bowls of it), and of course his old standby, broccoli. He's still averse to the broccoli stalks, but what kid isn't? Other new foods: Daddy's rotisserie chicken. Chicken sausage with spinach in it. Steak, although we are going very minimal on red meat because it's acidifying. We are all about alkalizing in this house now! This new interaction with food is such a contrast to his previous behavior.

I think it means he's not as mineral deficient as he used to be. I remember learning that zinc deficiency makes food taste bland and can be a major source of picky eating. I think ever since we started implementing Body Ecology principles and reducing the acid-forming foods (mainly too much protein) and ramping majorly up on the alkalizing foods, his system is absorbing nutrients from his food much more effectively.

Better digestion means improved mineral absorption, which means more hormone production, which means a better immune system, which means less toxicity, which means the vicious cycle is reversed, which means improved physical health. Improved physical health means a decrease or even elimination of autistic symptoms.

Ben seems to be coming out of himself. His eye contact and desire to interact with others are consistent these days. His story telling, the hallmark of his autism, as well as the hyper-giddiness that attends his stories, are still in full force. But Ben has choice now. He chooses not to tell stories at inappropriate times. He is learning to inquire whether the people around him want to do a story, rather than plunging in with no regard for the desires of others.

He told us this afternoon that he has a crush on a girl in his Hebrew-school class. He is practicing eating with his mouth closed. He did it really well at dinner tonight and at lunch. It's a Son-Rise Program group thing. We're all working on it and celebrating each other. It's important; his teacher told us last week that Ben's chewing with his mouth open is grossing out the other children. No kidding! Talk about critical social skills. His flexibility has markedly increased.

Sean and I are back to hoping, again, that Ben can and will fully recover. He's only ten. He's come light years in eight months, since we arrived in New York and he began at Otto Specht. Last year at this time, soccer? No way. temple? No way. Learning to have friends and having opportunities to do so? Not possible.

WEDNESDAY, APRIL 24, 2013

Ben just called me into his room. He yelled, "Mommy, you have to come here. I have to tell you something really serious and important about homeschool!"

I replied, mouth full of dinner, "Hold on, Ben, I'll be right there!"

"No, Mommy, it's really serious and important! You have to come!"

I ran over, eager to hear what he wanted to tell me.

Ben: I've been thinking about homeschool, and maybe it's not so good for me anymore. I mean, when I'm in my playroom, I'm told that I'm in charge of everything, but then I come out of homeschool and I think I'm still supposed to be in charge of everything, and that's a problem. What do you think, Mommy?

Me: [crying] Ben, I am profoundly impressed and touched by your wisdom and your self-awareness. Daddy and I have actually been talking about this very thing, but we never dreamed you would have the intelligence and understanding to think it yourself! I am so proud of you!

Right now Ben is saying to Alina, in the living room (away from me): Homeschool might be making me selfish instead of actually helping me. If I get my way now, then why shouldn't I always get my way? Something like that! I told Mommy what I thought—

Alina: [interrupting] She probably said it was crazy!

Ben: [grinning] No, she started crying, she was really happy when I told her! I'm going to ask my teachers what they think.

Addendum

Later, I tucked Ben in.

"Nigh-nigh, Ben."

"Good *night*! Nigh-nigh is for babies!"

THURSDAY, APRIL 25, 2013

One of Ben's teachers sent an email yesterday, describing how Ben's repetitively singing songs at school is annoying to the other children and alienating Ben from them. The incident Ben refused to discuss with me involved that dynamic, wherein Ben had gotten particularly upset after his classmates got annoyed with him for singing. Apparently Ben was also upset because the other children were having cookies that he couldn't have. Additionally, she wrote, "It seems to me that Ben is more present at the beginning of the morning on the days he bikes to school. He 'wanders' less with his feet during our morning exercises. I believe I also notice that his thoughts also wander somewhat less on those mornings. I would highly encourage the physical activity in the morning whenever possible."

Addressing the issue

After Ben's massive revelation last night about the fact that his Son-Rise Program might be teaching him to be selfish, I thought the moment was timely to discuss what had happened at school yesterday. Over breakfast, I brought up the fact that his teacher had sent me an email and that I would like to discuss it with him. "*No way! Never!*" yelled Ben. I let it go.

A few minutes later, I gently brought it back up again, starting with a celebration. "Ben, Ms. R told me she thinks you're doing better in school since you started riding your bike to school! Paying attention better, and more alert. Do you think she's right?" Ben looked up and nodded.

I continued. "Ms. R also said that you are singing the same lines of songs over and over again, and it is annoying the other children. I think this might be an example of what you were saying last night, about how your Son-Rise Program playroom at this point might be encouraging you to not think about what other people want or need. Can you imagine if Alina were singing the same song over and over and over again, and she knew you didn't like that song, how that might annoy you?"

Ben smiled and nodded. I continued, "Well, I think the other children are feeling that way when you sing your songs over and over again. A bit annoyed. And because they come from different experiences, they are not always able to be kind, and can sometimes even be mean. I think you should consider how they might feel when they ask you to stop singing, and you won't. Do you think you could try being more flexible with them?"

He seemed open to the idea. It will take him time, trial and error, two or three steps forward and one step backward, to develop this new capacity: awareness of others' wants and a willingness to comply with those wants, even at the expense, sometimes, of what feels good to him in that moment.

Where does autism end and free will begin for Ben? I'm not sure he can stop singing when he gets stuck; I have a suspicion, however, that a good portion of the time he is not actually stuck and could stop if he chose to do so.

At school, Ben plays the role of the goody-goody, completely and utterly, almost to the point of caricature. He loves school; he always wants to be kind to all; he wishes everyone would be loving with everyone. And he says these things all the time, much to the chagrin, entertainment, and, at times, annoyance of the other children. But at home, with Alina, he can be mean, taunting, and aggressive, sometimes pinching, biting, and slamming doors. It's almost as though his Bobby/A.M. story—the story in which Ben lives most of his waking mental life except when he is at school, and sometimes there as well, for all I know—depicts the two sides of him: a mean older boy (Bobby) juxtaposed with a goody-goody younger person (A.M.). No wonder he likes the story about Bobby and A.M. so much; it's about the two different sides of himself!

The fascinating question for me now is how do I support Ben in his new endeavor to be less self-centered? He calls it selfish, but I think it's actually about his focus being too much on himself, resulting in what looks like selfish behaviors. In other words, I don't think he's always deliberately selfish in the situations where he is inflexible and unwilling to cooperate with other people and their wishes. I think sometimes his purview simply does not go beyond what feels best and most comfortable (and possibly tolerable or even safe) to him in that particular moment. That's where the autism begins, and Ben's will ends, perhaps.

But the other children's experience of Ben is the same, regardless of whether it's deliberate selfishness or autism: he won't do what they want him to do. Or stop doing what they don't want him to do. So they become frustrated and reject or exclude him. Then he feels lost, unable to connect with them, and sad. So again, how do I leverage his newfound self-awareness of this problematic rigidity and relentless focus on his own will, while still celebrating his uniqueness and, at the same time, teaching him effective social navigation?

Help!

THURSDAY, APRIL 25, 2013

Earlier this week, I received a fascinating email from Ben's class teacher. Apparently the relationship with Max, the only other boy in his class, has improved, but the girls are intolerant of his extreme and, I think, not entirely false "goody-goodyness." The girls in his class don't understand that Ben was literally deprived of school, when he wanted and yearned desperately for it, for years. Now he has school, and he is infinitely happy, despite the problematic dynamics with the other children. I think his teacher needs to explain this to the children, so they can understand more easily why Ben is so high on school and such a "goody-goody."

FRIDAY, APRIL 26, 2013

Ben arrived home today from school, and I asked him how it went. He said, "Good. Something happened I'm eager to tell you about, but not now."

And it wasn't until just now, around 8 PM, on the car ride home from temple, that I asked Ben again what he was "eager" to share with me. He told me that at school today, while he was doing something pretend, Max came over and was trying to distract Ben, and so Ben went over to the girls to get away from Max. "Then," Ben explained, "I couldn't help myself and I started singing the verse. They got annoyed, Max came over, and the whole thing ended up in a mess."

I am amazed. Ben shared with total openness about a difficult school experience. He is aware I want to help him learn how to manage it, and he chose to tell me that the problem happened again. For an adult to be so open, able to check in, request support, and share about troubling moments in his or her life would be impressive. For a previously autistic ten-year-old? Remarkable.

I celebrated Ben for sharing with us about his experience at school today. Then I said, "Ben, this is exactly what we can work on together!" I asked him if he felt he *had* to do the verse or if he *wanted* to. I was trying to assess whether it was autism or feeling compelled to annoy the girls out of some underlying, ten-year-old relational dynamic. Ben replied, "I guess I got too focused. I was too focused on the verse." I asked him if he wanted to experiment with letting go of the verse when he's around them, to avoid these messes that keep happening. He said yes, he would.

I think it's the NAC together with biotin, and the alkalizing diet of Body Ecology that's helping. But mostly, I think it's Ben—growing, learning, and exploring his world: socially, emotionally, and courageously.

By the way, both children were exemplary in their behavior at temple this evening, even singing some of the Hebrew songs during the Shabbat service. Sean and I were brimming over with hope, gratitude, and pride (when we weren't snoring; both of us are way too tired).

SATURDAY, APRIL 27, 2013

Ben has decided he wants to be a hair stylist, makeup artist, and clothing designer. I am completely serious. He loves styling, drawing, designing, and color. Ben is also obsessed with certain girls—really into them. I don't think it's a sexual-identity thing; it doesn't seem to be, anyway, although that would just be one more parenting journey. I think he just loves hair styling, clothing design, and color!

Ben and I also use Ben's love for these female-gender-associated interests as a major basis for humor in our Bobby and A.M. stories, in which Ben Levin, the student, is actually a character in A.M.'s class. Bobby is, in fact, horrified that Ben, A.M.'s friend in the stories, has female-associated interests. A.M., on the other hand, has nothing but admiration and respect for Ben as a result of those same interests. Ben and I drive the hyperbole to the limit with new ideas to annoy Bobby. Bobby says things like, "What is Ben going to do next? Design ballet outfits? Become a personal shopper for kids? Style prom dresses?" We come up with these ideas until we are both in hysterics.

But actually, Ben really loves these interests. I, unfortunately, brought my own set of insecurities to the conversation about it this evening. Ben brought up again how excited he is about style, hair, makeup, and fashion. I'm not proud of my response.

Me: Ben, should I be concerned?

Ben: Why?

Me: Well these interests are typically very much girl interests.

Ben: Mommy, please don't say you're concerned. That makes me feel embarrassed.

Me: Ben, I didn't mean to say concerned. That was wrong. I really meant I am fascinated. [Can you say, *Mommy's a liar?*] I'm intrigued, because it's so wonderful and interesting that you love these things. You are going to be an artist! I am so proud of you! And you'll be so good at any of these fields, because you're so talented and you love them so much, that you'll make lots of money and you can help support the woman you eventually meet and marry!

It's just embarrassing, being so transparent and controlling. But Ben's progress thrills me: He's excited, and he's sharing his excitement with me!

WEDNESDAY, JUNE 5, 2013

Ben told me just now that if he isn't a fashion designer, he might like to be a writer. I told him that he is so gifted, he could do many things. "What are five of my gifts?" he asked. I replied:

1. The most important, he has a loving heart.
2. He is incredibly intelligent.
3. He is very handsome.
4. He writes wonderful stories.
5. He is extremely funny.

I told him I would love to see him be a teacher, if he doesn't end up a writer or designer. I like the idea of Ben connecting with other people in his chosen field versus the isolation typical of writers. He said he didn't think he'd be a great teacher, since he still struggles with long division. I explained he doesn't have to teach math; he could teach writing, for example. I told him about my friend, Jay, who is a professor of English and teaches about stories and literature and what they mean. I told Ben that Jay travels all over, learning about stories and ways to read them at conferences all over the world.

Ben then said, "Maybe I could start a school where we use stories to teach other things. Like I could tell a story and it would have math in it." "A story-telling school," I replied. "So it would be a school where stories are the vehicle for learning everything?" "Yes," he confirmed.

FRIDAY, JUNE 14, 2013

Yesterday was Ben's last day for this year at his new school. For the past several days, and possibly last week as well, Ben has been remote and nonresponsive. We went to an introduction to Cub Scouts meeting this past week, and Ben literally walked around in circles while the scoutmaster was trying to talk to him. He couldn't stay focused or stand still, for even a moment.

I have been upset about Ben's seeming regression into autistic symptoms, because (a) he has been remarkably nonautistic for months now and (b) I am still too hooked into the ups and downs of his recovery. But also, it seemed to come out of nowhere and that confused me. His food is great, we have made no changes recently in supplements, excluding some homeopathic remedies we ran out of that he has been off for a few weeks. But that alone shouldn't have created this much fogginess for him. There are no yeast symptoms (*e.g.*, circuiting, yeasty smell, hand flapping, irrational laughter), so yeast doesn't seem to be behind it. I theorized that perhaps it was an infection of some sort, gone undetected because of Ben's immunodeficiency disorder, which prevents Ben's body from showing the normal immune response in the presence of pathogenic bacteria or viruses. In other words, when there's an infection, Ben doesn't get a sore throat (immune response) or swollen glands (immune response). So an infection can be inside him, but we won't know it, and it can cause neurological problems.

But today he seemed to bounce back. He was bright eyed, interactive, and questioning in a very positive way. Today began the first day of Sillian School, Ben's imaginary school he has been engaged with for the past year. Ben has created lots of imaginary schools over the past two years. Sillian School takes place for one entire week at certain times of the year, outside of the normal, academic school year. Ben becomes very rigid about the dates of Sillian School. He has seemed to depend on Sillian School, and the other imaginary schools, as a way to cope with his not being in "real school" since the time he developed a desire to attend a real school and be with other children (*i.e.*, around two years ago). I haven't quite understood his need for Sillian School now that he is actually in a real school, other than simple obsession, which we believe is a symptom of Ben's PANDAS.

So this afternoon, Ben suddenly realized that the September week of Sillian School conflicts with our trip to Harry Potter World, and he became completely overwrought. Screaming, yelling, hysterical, crying, and even using physical force to try and get me and Alina to understand that the trip had to be canceled. His tantrum escalated into, "You hate me! You want me to die! I'm going to put a spear into myself and then you'll be happy! You've never loved me! You never wanted me!" I stayed calm, relaxed, and even-tempered as Ben went through his hysterics. At one point, Ben threatened Alina physically, and I stepped in. Otherwise, however, I maintained a Son-Rise Program attitude and did not judge Ben. I put him in his room, to the tune of "You hate me! You hate me!" He demanded that Alina answer a question related to the Disney trip, and once she did, he immediately became calm.

I asked him to come sit with me, so we could talk. Clearly ashamed of his earlier behavior, Ben said, "As long as we don't talk about before!" I agreed, and we sat down. I told him that I didn't understand why Sillian School was still so important to him, when he now had Otto Specht and a real class to be with. His face turned red, and he again became emotional, but this time it was not anger, but sadness. He explained to me that he needed to have a smaller brain, because the brain he has is too filled with ideas. I asked him if having so many ideas was painful or overwhelming, and he replied, "It's hard!"

He began to cry. My poor baby.

He continued, his face screwed up with the pain of what he was expressing, saying, "I think my imagination is too big. I have too much. I need you to ask God to make me a smaller brain!" I sat there in awe of what Ben was telling me. He confirmed, in so many words, that the incessant stories we have lived with since Ben's emergence from autism several years ago were enormously taxing for him, psychologically. "Perhaps," Ben offered, "we could start every day before 9 and then I wouldn't have time to tell the stories, and that would keep me from telling them!"

So he knows. Ben knows the stories are not right. He, too, doesn't want them anymore. They are a source of seeming agony to him, from the look on his face. I felt excited, like I was witnessing the incarnation of a soul. Ben was seeing himself, separating himself from his obsession, and understanding that the obsession was a problem for him.

I took a risk. I said, "Ben, when you can't stop thinking about something, the way you can't stop thinking about imaginative things you create? That's called obsession. Many, many kids have this problem." Ben's eyes widened. "Whaaaaaaaat?" he cried. "Yes, Ben. And there's something else. Obsession is one of the main things we see in children who have PANDAS. Do you remember Daddy and me telling you about PANDAS?" Ben nodded. "That's why we're going to the doctor, honey. He thinks if we do the pinch and the burn [Ben's name for the IVIG treatments], even though it's so yucky, that it will get rid of the PANDAS you have. And if we get rid of the PANDAS, we get rid of the obsession."

Ben looked stunned. His face smoothed out; the pain lines disappeared. He smiled and said, "That is a beautiful thing to hear."

Later I told him that not only kids have obsession (I thought the term "OCD" would be a little much for him to take in), but many grown-ups do, too. That blew him away. "Whaaaaaaaat???" he exclaimed for the second time. "Yes," I told him. "Some grown-ups are obsessed with washing their hands, so they wash them over and over again. Like twenty-five times. Some grown-ups are obsessed with the idea that they left the oven on at home, so they can't get out of the driveway to go somewhere because they have to come back and check the oven over and over again.

"Really, I'm not making this up!" I added, because Ben was clearly incredulous. The conversation was a moment of revelation for me, that Ben's stories are a source of such pain for him, and a moment of enlightenment for Ben, about the nature of obsession and the hope for successful treatment through IVIG. I also believe that when one is aware of the goal of a given intervention, such as IVIG, and one desires that goal intensely, the power of the mind and spirit to move toward that goal is very real. So I want Ben to know what we are trying to do with IVIG and to focus his will and spirit on succeeding.

After all was said and done, Ben returned to complete his day of Sillian School. The last class is "diarying." I wondered what he would write about.

As Ben was writing, I was taking notes on the conversation. He looked over, and I told him I was just writing down what we had talked about before I forgot it all. He came over and read a bit of what I had written. He smiled and asked, "Who are you writing to exactly, Mommy?" "It's my book, honey!" I replied.

Ben paused and said, firmly, "I do not want you to publish this to the public!"

Yikes, I thought. There go the royalties!

"Why not, Ben?" Alina asked. I knew the answer before Ben said it.

"Because it's embarrassing!"

"But Ben," I asked, "what if other children have this problem, and we've found an answer for you, and those other families need to know this answer, and we would be helping so many people?"

"Well," Ben looked stumped for a moment. "Why can't you just call them?"

"Because books reach so many more people, all over the world, Ben! We can help families all over the world!"

"Well, it's still too embarrassing, and I don't want you to do it."

"Okay," I replied. I'll deal with all that later, I thought to myself.

One final note. As Ben was diarying a few moments ago, he suddenly blurted out:

"Mommy, I have another piece of truth I just realized."

"What's that, Ben?"

"You can't spend every day you're not in school in your imagination."

"Why not, Ben?"

"Because your parents might have other plans for you." Like going to Harry Potter World, for example?

SATURDAY, JUNE 15, 2013

I wasn't sure what exactly Ben took away from the conversations yesterday about obsession and IVIG and the rest. But this morning, at breakfast with Sean, Ben suddenly blurted out, "Mommy told me that PANDAS will help me stop having too many stories!" I gently corrected him. "I think you mean to say that the PANDAS is causing you to have too many stories, and the IVIG will help you get rid of that problem?" "Yes!" Ben confirmed. He seemed genuinely excited and hopeful.

I guess it went in.

WEDNESDAY, JUNE 19, 2013

From Sean

"This morning at six, when Ben got out of bed, I heard, 'Where's Daddy?' After he found me, he gave me his night-light and said, 'Daddy, I think I'm too old for a night-light.' I thanked Ben for telling me, and he said, 'I just wanted you to know.'

"My supposedly autistic son is back to being 'supposedly' autistic. Maybe it really was because school was ending, but he is not the same person he was three or four days ago. He is very present, engaging in conversation, being flexible, doing things he hasn't done before, like eat spinach leaves and, at my request, help carry groceries from the car to the kitchen!

"Anyway, my supposedly autistic son just (1) told me what he was thinking and (2) 'wanted' me to know what it was he was thinking. It wasn't about me being in the right place at the right time. It was my son having a thought, that he's too old for night-lights, and then thinking, 'I Want To Tell Daddy!' For parents of neurotypical children, this may not seem to be a big deal, but for us, with a son like Ben, it's a blessing.

"I appreciate that it occurred on Father's Day. I think Father's Day is a very foolish day, right after Mother's Day, but that is a rant for another day. Today, nine months after picking up my family and moving, after changing my career so I still work for the same employer but can never get promoted, after incurring more financial hardship, my son took a couple of minutes and told me it was worth it. My son sought me out because he wanted to share a thought. And that truly is the best Father's Day gift I've ever had."

SATURDAY, JUNE 22, 2013

Thursday and Friday of this week were Ben's second round of IVIG. We drank a lot more water both days than last round, since last round he vomited hugely the second night. So this time, no headache and no vomiting. This morning, however, Ben woke up and was tense. Yesterday, in fact, at the procedure, he was extremely anxious and rigid. The nurse practitioner at the clinic said that was not a typical response to IVIG. Anyway, this morning, I decided it might be good for Ben not to have his usual half of a green apple to start the day. I am wanting to ease into the Body Ecology full-throttle protocol, now that we have successfully introduced many new recipes and I think Ben can handle letting go of some of his old standby foods.

Big mistake. I messed up his morning routine by saying no to his usual apple, and he lost his mind. As Alina described, Ben went "mad house. Worse than mad house!" He became furious, hitting and lashing out, screaming and calling all of us mean names. It lasted about two hours, on and off. Sean gave Ben a capsule of activated charcoal, and soon after he was calm, somewhat remorseful even, and placid the remainder of the day.

I don't know if this reaction was die-off from the IVIG killing off some bad-guy antibodies or what. I have totally no idea. I made cacao chocolate this week, and Ben had five or six pieces yesterday, but it's made with stevia, coconut oil, and raw cacao butter and powder—that is, no yeast-causing ingredients. He did eat an entire box of strawberries the night before, and he also had strawberries (a small bowl) and a hamburger and salad at a regular restaurant last night after the procedure, so there may have been a reaction to one of those foods. But I don't think so. I have not seen Ben quite so acutely out of control in a very long time. I think he was beyond exhausted from the two six-hour days of transfusions, not to mention the four-plus hours of driving both days. And the activated charcoal seemed to have done the trick, which makes me think there were some sort of toxins that needed a speedy escort out of his body.

Camp starts Monday.

SUNDAY, JUNE 23, 2013

Tonight, as I was tucking Ben in after reading our nightly chapter of Harry Potter (we are on Book Five), Ben asked me, "Which of the four Hogwarts houses do you think I would be in?" I replied, instantly, "Gryffindor. You're so brave, Ben, I don't even have to think about it!" "Oh," he replied, nonplussed. "That's my third choice. I'm not really very brave. I would like to be in Hufflepuff, and if not, then Ravenclaw, because I'm so intelligent. Do you think I would do well in Ravenclaw?" Pleased and amused as always by my ten-year-old's honest observation of his own strengths and weaknesses, I replied, "Well I think I see you differently than you see you. I often hear you say you are nervous about doing certain things, and yet you do them anyway, and that to me is bravery. You are fiercely intelligent, so Ravenclaw would be good. Why would you want to be in Hufflepuff? You don't seem so, I don't know, puffy!"

Ben replied, "I don't like facing battles and that sort of thing. It's embarrassing. Hufflepuffs enjoy a simple life, and that's what I want. Working hard, doing good things. I think that's the best." My own little Buddha! I laughed and said, "Wow, that's amazing, Ben. So you don't want everyone looking at you, and talking about you, like if you were in the middle of adventures and famous for them?" He nodded. I continued. "It's also interesting, Ben, because I don't think Alina feels that way. I think she likes to do adventures and be in the middle of stuff."

Ben grinned. Then he asked, "What do you like, Mommy?" I grinned back and replied, "I don't know, Ben. I used to always want to be in the middle of things, with everyone looking at me. But then I realized that the things that made me the happiest had nothing to do with any of that. It was more about you and Daddy and Alina. I'm happiest when we're reading Harry Potter or eating dinner outside on the deck or talking to you right now. So it's confusing. A part of me still wants the big, showy stuff, but the real part of me knows that's not what is the really big stuff. I honestly haven't quite figured it out yet.

"But Daddy's like you, Ben. He likes the simple life: being with family, working hard, all that. I'm more the other. But like I said, I'm a little confused." I loved the rest of the conversation:

Ben: What's the Mommy part of me, and what's the Daddy part of me?

Me: The Daddy part of you is your simplicity, your understanding that hard work and family are the real things in life. The Daddy part of you is your sarcastic sense of humor and your brilliant mind. You're really strong and athletic, and you get that from Daddy, too, and definitely not from me. Your sense of order and your abilities in math. Your shyness, too, you get that from Daddy. I used to be shy, but I'm really not now. But Daddy gets that way sometimes.

Ben: What are the Mommy parts of me?

Me: Well, also your sarcastic sense of humor! Also your smarts.

Ben: But what do I get that's just you?

Me: Ben, you get your creativity from me. [Huge smile from Ben] I am always creating things. I never stop. And your musicality. And perhaps your honesty, your directness, and straightforwardness, although that's Daddy, too.

Ben: Who did I get my good looks from?

HA!

Me: Well, that's probably your Dad. I'm good-looking, too, don't get me wrong. But Daddy's got a star quality with his looks that you have. But you got my eyes, thank God, you got my eyes. And my mouth!

And with that, my beautiful boy leaned back on his pillow, ready for sleep.

He's nervous about camp starting tomorrow. He really wants to make friends but doesn't feel he knows how. I told him, just before turning off the light tonight, that I know he's nervous about making friends tomorrow at camp, that I chose this particular camp because they will help him to make friends, and that I would remind his counselors that he needs some help with that. He smiled and looked relieved. Such a sweet boy. The children had to fill out a form for their counselors to bring to camp tomorrow. One of the questions asked, "Do you have any concerns about coming to camp?" Ben responded, "Making new friends." The following question was, "What would you like your counselors to know about you?" Ben wrote, "I like being creative."

Ben and Alina. Rainbows in my heart.

MONDAY, JUNE 24, 2013

Ben's first day went well

Quick update: Ben had a nice day at camp today. He said it was a little fun! I asked him why it was only a little fun, and he replied it just was. I asked him if there were any kids there he wanted to be friends with, and he said no. So I don't know if he just played by himself or what. But I have to let go. He's there, he's learning, and he's practicing. And

I'm praying! I think he feels great to be doing what "normal" kids do—go to camp. He certainly looked it today.

TUESDAY, JUNE 25, 2013

An email from Granpa

Susan,

Your conversation with Ben, about the "Mommy and Daddy parts" of Ben, was remarkable in so many ways. The self-awareness and thoughtfulness Ben displayed would be amazing in anyone, much less a ten-year-old kid with his particular problems. You and Sean are entitled to feel very proud.

Dad

WEDNESDAY, JUNE 26, 2013

Ben seems to be getting on very well at camp, despite the long days—with activities running nonstop from 9 AM until 4 PM—and hot weather right now as well. Today they had to choose from a selection of "hobbies," and Ben chose skits, which of course requires total interaction with others! He said it was fun and that he chose it because he's good at it. Ben is actually very good on stage. He has a resonant voice and loves being in front of people.

He also mentioned waiting in line for the bathroom at one point *with his friend, Luke,* both of them irritated that the younger kids ahead of them were taking so long. Apparently they tried to distract themselves by talking about something, but to no avail; they both had to go so badly! They had to wait for *three whole minutes,* Ben told me. "Everyone in Group H is so immature!" he remarked. Also, yesterday he apparently had a nice conversation with a girl named Caroline in his group about books they are currently reading and why they liked them. His counselor told me about the conversation, and Ben said it was a really nice time.

Ben is exhausted by the end of the camp day and reacts badly to Alina, who is also exhausted and provocative. Tonight Ben absolutely lost it in a rage about something—I forget what—and then an hour later was wild with laughter, in a state of hysteria over a joke about one of his made-up stories. Everyone's on overdrive from camp.

Later, however, when we were reading Harry Potter, I wanted to skip a section in the book when one of Harry's teachers tortures him. I hated the section when I read it the first time, and as I actually act out the story, I really didn't want to do that portion. But Ben would not let me skip any of the chapter. He became furious and insisted that I read it, although it felt emotionally painful for me to do so, and I said so. I compromised by saying I would read it very quickly. Ben replied, "You can read it so fast we can't even hear you; that's fine." I understood then that he was just stuck, and I said to him, "Do you feel like you're not going to be okay if I don't read it all?" He nodded his head. "So then this isn't something you can control, sweetheart. I get it; it's the autism. No problem." I read the chapter, and it was okay.

I don't know if I should talk to him so freely about autism, but I like to do so, to demystify it for him and also let him know I'm aware he can't control the rigidity when it hits him. He is still extremely rigid at times. When, for example, I told the children that they could do an extra week of camp in July if they wanted to, but they would have to miss a day because we will be coming home from the mountains, Ben was adamant that missing even one day—even *half* of one day—meant he couldn't do any camp that week.

But he's learning a lot at camp. I'm so pleased he's there, learning, stretching, and getting strong modeling from other children with better social skills.

WEDNESDAY, JULY 3, 2013

Last night, Ben spent his first night away from home without any family. He went on an overnight camping trip with his group at camp. He was out of his mind with excitement, madly running up to children in his group, singing, "And tonight's gonna be a good night, and tonight's gonna be a good-good night!" He's still learning about personal space, but I felt so happy for him.

The other night, I had asked Ben, "How do you feel about going on the camping trip?" Without hesitation, Ben responded, "I'm a little nervous. But I know it will be good." I was impressed, as usual, with his authenticity—and his faith. He chooses to expect good things will come, and even when life knocks him down, he always finds a way home to happiness. Even with the things he wants the most, such as friends, he's patient. We talked the next day, and I said, "You know, Ben, this is your first time totally away from us, without any of your family there!" He replied, "I know. I'm ten." He beamed with pride.

Last night, while Ben was on the trip, Sean and I tried to be mature, trusting, and excited for Ben's adventure, but instead we were both terrified. When one of his counselors called during the day to say Ben had dropped his lunch and could I please bring something over (they hadn't left yet for the camp-out), I nearly had a heart attack, thinking they were calling because Ben had freaked out.

Then this morning, after depositing Alina with her bunk, I strolled over to Ben's area, where I knew he and his bunkmates would be preparing for Day Two of this week's adventure: a three-hour sailing trip. I saw one of the counselors, Emily, outside the room. She grinned and gave me a huge thumbs-up. Apparently Ben had a great time last night, and when he got up this morning, Ben had told her he was relieved to have made it through the night. Emily asked me if I wanted her to send Ben out to me, and I said, "Why don't you just tell him his mom's here to drop off his little sister, and did he want to come out and say hello?" Emily went inside and a few moments later emerged, saying, "No, he doesn't want to say hi."

Good for you, kiddo! And, of course, a little sad for me. Naturally, I felt disappointed. But that's unimportant. Ben is excited to be separate and independent. He knows we trust him now. Significantly, I wasn't surprised that he didn't want to see me. As he said, he's ten. And he's improving. Later, I happened to look out the window and see a clear, blue sky. I thought to myself, "Wow, I wonder if Ben's out there sailing, looking up at the sky, and feeling like a real boy."

WEDNESDAY, JULY 3, 2013

Ben had a wonderful time on his camp-out and sailing trip! I picked him up, and he ran to me, desperate for a hug. I was glad I hadn't forced myself on him this morning, when he was enjoying his independence. He loved the sailing and told us at dinner it was because he loved just hanging out with his friends. I asked him if he shared the crackers I had packed for him and his friends (raw but store-bought so perhaps, I thought, a little appealing to other kids). He responded in the negative. "The children were having marshmallows. I didn't even offer the crackers; I knew they wouldn't want them." Smart kid.

He was desperate for a story, launching into it on the car ride home from camp. Who could blame him? Interactive story telling for Ben is like excellent television shows for me: a necessary escape. Ben was "on" for two days straight, with no family, no outward supports, no stories, no nothing—just himself and the inner strength he has developed over the past six years.

Tonight, I asked Ben how he liked the corn on the cob they served on the trip. It's Ben's favorite food, and he has not been able to have it for over five years. He told me he loved it and, furthermore, that he asked his counselors "to report any autistic behavior that came afterwards, in case he wasn't able to digest it properly." Boy, does the child listen. I asked him if any autistic behavior had been "reported," and he said no. I told him I wasn't surprised. It was a great time. The only way out is through—scaredy-cat parents and all.

SUNDAY, JULY 7, 2013

For the past week, Ben has been up and down. We are seeing some old rigidity, some tantruming, some giddy laughter, and some circuiting. Yeast? Ben himself suggested to me two or three days ago that we should take out "all the new foods for a week, and then just add one at a time, and see which is the problem." He understands so much. So again I become a sleuth, trying to understand what has happened to send him back into some autistic behaviors. Too much yeasty food that I didn't know was yeast-causing? Overstimulating week? IVIG backfiring? Sean reminded me two weeks after the first round, last month, we saw some intensely autistic behavior, Ben was literally walking in circles at the Cub Scout intro meeting. It's such an ongoing process. We'll narrow the diet again and see how he does.

MONDAY, JULY 8, 2013

Ben presented with a lot of yeasty behaviors again today. Circuiting, hysterical laughter, constant nonresponsiveness, and, most upsetting, rage-filled outbursts when he could not obtain or achieve what he wanted, swiftly followed by lucid and calm explanations. Almost like he's two different people.

Round and round, round and round, and round and round. "Systemic yeast infection" is the subject and premise of Donna Gates's Body Ecology Diet work, and Ben is textbook. We get better, make so much progress, and then whoops—down the rabbit hole again. Ben hasn't lost any of the gains. They just go into hiding when yeast rears its ugly head. No offense, God, but I'm sick of character building!

TUESDAY, JULY 9, 2013

Ben seems better today. Also, I read an article on salicylates in food, which talked about chlorine in the summer for immuno-compromised kids and what it does to them. And that we can use Epsom-salts baths and cream to help detox the chlorine.

Yay, Mommy.

Yay, research.

Yay, persistence!

THURSDAY, JULY 18, 2013

This week, Ben went on an overnight canoe trip. When I asked him how it went, he said, "Great! But canoeing is hard and boring." I asked him what his favorite part of the trip was, and he told me it was looking at the moon after the campfire.

I'm thrilled Ben is having childhood experiences like this. He deserves it.

SUNDAY, JULY 21, 2013

This afternoon, Ben and Alina got into a small fight. Ben threatened to pinch Alina. I sent him to his room. I came in to talk. I asked him why he was being so aggressive and grouchy lately. Did he think it was the new food? "I don't know," he answered. After a few moments, Ben said to me, "I think sometimes this has been a more miserable year than I've ever had before. Do you think the number thirteen is unlucky beyond Friday the 13th? I mean, do you think the year 2013 could be unlucky too? Because this year has been so much harder than my other years."

Me: How so, Ben? Do you mean the stuff with Max?

Ben: Yes, but no. I mean more inside of me, I'm grouchy, and I get so rigid.

It's fascinating because he is now so self-aware. Ironically, he doesn't realize just how rigid he was when he was younger and in the throes of autism.

I paused, considering how to respond.

Me: Ben, I don't think thirteen is unlucky, even Friday the 13th. That's just superstition. Here's the thing. This year, you turned ten, and a lot of things happened. You started being more grown-up, realizing you are your own person, not just an extension of me and Daddy and Alina. Your body started to change, which meant you had a lot more "grrrrrrr!" feelings inside of you, which is normal for a boy. And also, you started school, a real school, with other children. Ben, when you were little, you were at preschool, and it was different.

Ben: You mean, because I was just a little kid who didn't know things?

Me: No, because you were autistic. You were with other children, but you didn't interact with them. You didn't have friends, like you have now. You were there, but you couldn't reach out and really play with other kids. Now, you don't have that problem anymore. You want friends. You're in school with other children, and you're having to work a lot harder. You're making a lot of mistakes, because that's what we do when we're learning something new. You're also having a lot of successes. And that's awesome. And Daddy and I are so proud of you. The other thing is, from when you were two or three years old until just a few years ago, you had autism. And that means you couldn't learn a lot of things that other children do in those years. So you missed a lot of lessons having to do with making friends. So now you're catching up. And it's hard, because you're behind.

Ben continued to consider my words.

Me: But you're doing it! And Daddy and I have no doubt at all that you are going to catch all the way up and have an awesome girlfriend, an awesome bar mitzvah, and an awesome life. But this part is, as you are feeling, hard.

Ben nodded.

Me: Ben, it means so much to me that you can say these things to me. That's the most important thing. Whatever you feel, let it out. Don't keep it inside of you. That's the best thing.

He came out of his room and went and apologized to Alina. "Alina, I'm sorry I got mad and tried to interrupt your book. I didn't deserve it; it's your book."

Alina, absorbed in a computer game, responded, "It's fine, Ben. No problem."

SATURDAY, AUGUST 3, 2013

Sean and I just got home from a four-day getaway, without the kids, up in the Berkshires. Last night, when we called to say good night, I asked Ben and Alina if they were excited to see us today. Ben yelled, "I'm so excited I am going to kiss the phone!" Then, because Alina talked over him, Ben wasn't sure I'd heard him, and he repeated, "I'm so excited I'm going to kiss the phone, Mommy!"

Today we arrived home around one o'clock. Ben was waiting outside for us in the driveway. As we pulled in, his face lit up with joy. He ran around to my side of the van, and when I opened the door, he ran over and gave me the world's biggest hug, kiss, and smile. I said, "I missed you, Ben!" He replied, "I missed you too, Mommy! My pretty Mommy, I'm so glad you're home!"

I started Ben tonight on a six-day Oxypowder colon cleanse. Poor baby. Seven capsules every night, and he will be spending a good amount of time in the loo. But it's a gentler way to cleanse than all the enemas. He goes through so much. Everything we've done. Thank God he knows it's because I love him.

SUNDAY, AUGUST 4, 2013

Deep thoughts

I just came from putting the children to sleep. Sean is in Boston, and his father, Morris, whom the children call "Zayde" in Yiddish, is in the hospital. It's worrisome; they are running tests to try and figure out why he has been in pain lately. Earlier this evening, I told the children Zayde was in the hospital for tests and that we needed to pray for him but that we think he will be fine. Ben said he was glad to hear it. As I tucked Ben in tonight, he leaned up and stroked my hair. "When you die," he suddenly remarked, "I will save a piece of your hair, for a memory. I don't mean to talk about you dying; it just occurred to me." Ben used to talk about my "yellow hair," when he was smaller. He's always liked it.

Me: That's okay, Ben. I don't mind talking about it. I'm not afraid of death.

Ben [without a pause]: Do you think we have more than one life?

Me: Yes, I do.

Ben: So do I. Alina doesn't.

Me: Maybe she just doesn't like to focus on what's next, since she's so fully *here*, in this life. But to me, it's the only thing that makes sense.

Ben: Mmm-hmm.

Me: I think what stays with us forever is love and the connections we choose to make in each lifetime. We don't lose those; they are always there.

That was it. Reincarnation and the meaning of life—at nigh-nighs.

I love it that Ben considers these issues and chooses to discuss them with me. What a transformation from the isolated and seemingly uninterested boy he used to be. He couldn't act on it before, but today, having 'gotten to know' my son for the past four-plus years, I am sure that Ben was always, always interested in us. Today, having "met and gotten to know" my son for the past four-plus years, I am *sure* that Ben was always, always interested in us, regardless of his inability to act on it.

Ben the receptionist
Ben decided about two weeks ago that he really likes answering the phone. He does it really well, politely and audibly.

Where have all the mommies gone?
Final note for tonight. I have transformed, somehow, during my four-day-vacation absence from Ben, from Mommy to *Mom*. Every time Ben spoke to me or referred to me today, I was no longer Mommy. *Mom*. Ben is claiming his almost-eleven-year-old status.

I *think* I'm okay with that.

TUESDAY, AUGUST 20, 2013

Ben is writing a book, based loosely on Harry Potter. Like Harry Potter, there are seven volumes in the series. Like Harry Potter, the books' themes are basically good versus evil and children in a school battling evil together. Unlike Harry Potter, the book is about a Jewish kid named Gabriel Garnet, who attends a school with twelve dormitories—each named after one of the twelve tribes of Israel, and whose final chapter will culminate in Gabriel's *bar mitzvah*.

This morning, I asked Ben, "Why did you run off ten copies of your Gabriel Garnet book?" Ben replied, "Because I want my book to be really popular!"

On another note: earlier today, Ben said to me, "I love having you in my life!"

THURSDAY, AUGUST 22, 2013

Later, I spoke with Alina and told her when Danny and I were kids, and I had lots of friends, I felt guilty that Danny had none. "Like Ben?" she asked. I answered in the affirmative and told her I didn't want her to feel that way, guilty because she has friends and Ben doesn't. "I don't," she replied calmly.

FRIDAY, AUGUST 23, 2013

A conversation with Ben today:

Ben: Sometimes I think T. (a friend at school) has even more trouble making friends than I do.

Me: Yes, Ben, because she isn't even aware—

Ben: Yes, she doesn't realize.

Me: But, Ben, you do realize, and I think instead of isolating—do you know what that that means? Choosing to be alone to avoid other people. Instead of isolating, you should *watch* other children and see how they make friends, watch them to learn. Don't go and read; watch them. You weren't with kids for a long time, so you need to learn from them.

Ben: Mmm-hmm.

MONDAY, SEPTEMBER 9, 2013

Today Ben returned for his second year at Otto Specht and had a great day. He was excited to be back, and since the other boy in his class—who became exceedingly aggressive to Ben and the other children in Ben's class last year—was out sick today, the first day was easier than expected. He is exhausted but cheerful.

Currently, Ben:

- Sets the table at meals

- Gets out his vitamins as well as mine
- Puts his clothing out the night before school (just started this)
- Cleans up his toys after dinner, with support
- Is able to use the phone and has regular conversations with grandparents and former au pairs and other friends, when he's not too tired
- Reads voraciously, mostly books that are too young for him: chapter books, whose simple plot lines and characters he then uses to generate his own variations on their themes
- Has written a seven-section chapter book of his own, based loosely on Harry Potter, the story of Jacob's sons in the Bible, and science fiction themes
- Constantly expresses his feelings with eloquence, authenticity, and a keen desire to connect and be heard
- Has friends and is learning to be a good friend
- Poops every day
- Is still more tired than he should be
- Goes to bed around 8 and is up often before 5 AM
- Rides his bike to school most days
- Has massive word-retrieval problems that cause him to stammer and stutter and repeat words, which interferes terribly with his social interactions, especially with new friends or situations
- Eats the Body Ecology Diet and takes a reasonable amount of supplements, but not the avalanche of pills he used to when we did the DAN! protocol
- Seems extremely young for his age and profoundly naive, unsophisticated, and even uninterested in certain, basic social rules and dynamics

SUNDAY, SEPTEMBER 1, 2013

In March 2009, Sean and I attended a Son-Rise Program course. During that week, we made friends with a number of parents. At the end of the week, brimming with hope, we all agreed to meet at Disneyworld with our "recovered kids" in 2013. Why 2013? A random choice.

Tomorrow morning, at 11:13, our family—including Ben—will actually, miraculously, depart for Disney! Actually, we'll depart for Universal's Islands of Adventure, which hosts the Wizarding World of Harry Potter—the apex of existence for my children. (We are now on Book Six of the seven-book series. I read some every night to the children, and we are all enchanted.) We knew back in 2009 at that course that what we promised each other was possible, but for it to actually happen? Seemed too good to be true. Yet now it's happening. We are still in touch with some of those parents, though the Disney plan has not been discussed since our hopeful promise to each other over four years ago.

At any rate, tomorrow morning we will hop on over to Newark International Airport and JetBlue down to Orlando. One afternoon of hotel fun (*e.g.*, big fancy beds, pools, kids' activities room), one day at SeaWorld, one day at Harry Potter World (explosions, fireworks, and so forth), and then home on an early flight on Thursday morning. Short, sweet, and inconceivable before now.

I'm not even scared. If Ben has a hard time for some reason, if the children scrap, if Sean and I bicker—who cares?! We are living life. We are going to Harry Potter World!

MONDAY, SEPTEMBER 2, 2013

We made it! We are in Orlando. But what a day we had. Our flight was delayed for two and a half hours, but the children were wonderful. They did not complain; they did not whine; they sat patiently for two hours and ate their lunches, played on the computer, and laughed with each other. We finally arrived at our beautiful hotel, the Parc Soleil, at 7:45 PM, having left our home in New York at 9 this morning. The children had eaten only a few turkey hot dogs since three o'clock, and we were all tired and hungry. Yet neither child had a tantrum, exploded, or misbehaved. Sean and I were actually the irritable ones!

So now the children are asleep, and Sean is at Whole Foods, picking up things like digestive enzymes, flax oil, kefir, and millet. Hey, we wouldn't be the Levins if we could do food at Disney like a normal family! And Ben wouldn't be progressing out of autism, either.

What a minute! Did I say Disney? *I meant Harry Potter World!*

TUESDAY, SEPTEMBER 3, 2013

Today didn't go so well. First of all, I had a terrible night's sleep, and as soon as I got up, I realized I had a stomach flu.

Ben also woke up sick. The children went to the pool and children's recreation room for the morning, and then Alina and our au pair, Tim, went to SeaWorld. Sean stayed home to take care of Ben so I could rest. Around 3:00, Sean took Ben to Barnes & Noble, where Ben read the same chapter books that he reads back at home every day. Sean came home looking deeply pained but wouldn't tell me why. "I can't right now," he said.

At 5:00, Sean left to meet Alina and Tim at SeaWorld for a 5:30 showing of a movie about killer whales. Five minutes ago, we spoke on the phone. Sean was crying. "While we were at the bookstore, I called Alina. She told me she went on a ride. She said it was the scariest ride of her life, and she almost got off, but she didn't, she did the ride, and she is so proud of herself. And I have a disabled son, and I missed it. I missed Alina doing her ride. I sat in a Barnes & Noble with my son and watched him read books. And I missed it. I don't care about Harry Potter World; I love SeaWorld. And I spent the whole day missing it."

My husband rarely cries. Earlier today, when I was in self-pity that the family couldn't be together at SeaWorld, he offered the perspective that God knew Ben couldn't handle two days of theme parks, and so this was actually a good solution. I kind of bought it; all I really care about is Harry Potter World anyway. I felt sad that we were split up, but it wasn't Ben's autism that caused it; we were just sick.

But I can see how Sean would interpret the day as one more situation where he was missing out on an experience that other fathers get to have with their daughters—and that Sean wanted to have with Alina. Frankly, Ben is sitting next to me, muttering to himself, spinning stories, writing them out onto paper to empty the flood of ideas constantly pouring into his mind, asking me for numbers that correspond to characters, and it's hard. It's autism, and it's not a typical vacation day in Orlando. Autism is mysterious. Ben seems fine some moments, but he is still fragile. We get by, but it's not always easy.

TUESDAY, SEPTEMBER 3, 2013

Sean came home from SeaWorld feeling much better. For my part, I spent the last few hours doing stories with Ben and thinking, "Is this ever going to change?"

WEDNESDAY, SEPTEMBER 4, 2013

Harry Potter World was great. Everyone had fun, everyone behaved well, and amazingly, all our expectations were fulfilled. Ben went on a roller coaster *four times*. I was surprised. I never dreamed he would love an experience where you are so out of control and subject to physical intensity. But he has become more fearless, less anxious, and more able to handle sensory experiences.

Alina loved the shops, drank Butterbeer, bought Zonko's Joke Shop toys, and loved Honeyduke's—what kid wouldn't! Tonight she was in heaven with her Extendable Ears.

We are packing and will be up with the dawn to catch our flight back to New York. Today gave us a treasure trove of new memories.

This evening we celebrated Rosh Hashanah in our hotel room with our dinner of leftovers, and celebrated the year that is ending and the year that is starting. *Shana tova!* Harry Potter World—a magnificent way to begin the Year 5773.

Yesterday was difficult, but today was great.

Last year was difficult. The new year will be *filled with blessings*.

SUNDAY, SEPTEMBER 29, 2013

Ben's favorite new song is "Firework," by Katy Perry. He said to me just now, "Mom, do you know what my favorite line in 'Firework' is? It goes, 'Do you know that there's still a chance for you?' It fills me with so much hope."

Hope. There's a concept.

We just endured one more round of IVIG to treat Ben's PANDAS. Ben had a panic attack when the nurse attempted to insert the IV. It lasted about forty-five minutes. At the end, I excused myself to a small side room and sobbed. Ben heard me and came over. He looked heartbroken and said, "Mom, I'll do it. I don't want to see you cry." I replied, "Ben, it's okay. I just want you to be healthy, and I'm worried if you don't do the IVIG—I just don't know what we'll do." I wasn't trying to guilt-trip, but I was absolutely wrecked. He repeated, "I'll do it, Mom."

So we went back into the nurse's station, and he tried again. Again he panicked and couldn't do it. He went rigid. I said, "It's okay, Ben. It's okay. We'll figure something else out." But I was welling up again, and Ben said, "No. I'm going to do it." This time he did. Once the IV was in, Ben relaxed, and the rest of the day went well. Since returning home, Ben has vacillated between lucid and fog. He's also exhausted from the procedure and traveling to the clinic. He's not the only one.

Ben just read this entry and remarked, "Well maybe crying is sometimes a good thing! When I saw you crying, it made me decide to do the IVIG!" Ben used to hate when I would write about him in my blog. He wanted his privacy. Now he doesn't seem to mind.

FRIDAY, OCTOBER 4, 2013

Ben asked a boy to play basketball with him at school today. They played. Ben also had several friends over this evening and was friendly and interactive the whole evening. He is doing better and connecting more. IVIG helps—a lot. I just don't know if its effects will last.

TUESDAY, OCTOBER 8, 2013

As this new school year is unfolding, Sean and I are witnessing yet another change in Ben. Changes like this are subtle, and almost missable, because they happen so organically that their presence seems just another part of life. But seen from the proper perspective, they are meaningful and heartening. This change is in his sudden wealth of social opportunities and blossoming friendships. When we lived in Boston, I turned myself inside out for years trying to create social opportunities for Ben. I searched for playdates, homeschooling groups, anything that might give Ben practice and a feeling of connection to other children. Everything failed. Playdates were limited, first-date-nothing-more endeavors. Our homeschool group petered out within months, and though friendships were established through that group, the actual time spent with other children was fractional. Perhaps it wasn't the right time.

Flash forward a year and a half to the present, where Ben's weeks are now replete with social situations. First, he is in school from 8:30 until 2:45 every day. He has become a cherished and beloved member of his school, whose population of fifteen-plus children has, this year, successfully achieved a loving cohesion that is clearly nurturing all of the children. Twice a week we have playdates at our home with friends from his school, whose working parents need a place for their children to hang out after school. Tuesday afternoons and Sunday mornings, Ben also has Hebrew school, where he joins a group of seven other children for two hours. On Sunday mornings, Ben has tutoring, temple choir, then Hebrew class. Ben's receiving tutoring not because he is remedial, but because he is so strong that his teachers wish to give him advanced training. "He *will* be the first formerly-autistic rabbi; you wait and see!" said his Hebrew teacher recently.

Ben made a new and very adorable friend at Hebrew school, a little girl in his class. She and Ben are chums, save seats for each other, and sing together in the temple's junior choir. The little girl's family lives in the next town over from ours. Last Sunday, I was sitting in the temple library with Alina, and Ben came tearing in, yelling, "Mom! Come quick! Mom! Come quick!" I hurriedly got up, and followed Ben up the stairs, to find the little girl and her mother waiting for us. "Mom, can we have a playdate sometime?" Ben inquired, almost dancing with excitement.

Later, Ben asked me, "Mom, have I ever done so much work to be someone's friend?" "No, Ben, I don't think so!" I replied, impressed as ever with Ben's self-perception. "But it helps that she's so cute!" I added, and Ben's face exploded in smiles. Ben might have a little girlfriend.

Ben is also still working on *Gabriel Garnet*, his seven-volume series about a Jewish boy who saves a bunch of good guys from a bunch of bad guys. Ben's first volume, *The Visitor's Secret*, has eleven chapters and is actually quite well written, especially for an almost-eleven-year-old. Ben and I designed the cover together, including a blurb we co-wrote:

> *Gabriel Garnet is really excited. He is starting Hebrew school soon. Meanwhile the knights of Clah, the King of Rynin, home of the wicked people, are kidnapping Jews for slaves. Little by little does Gabriel know it's up to him and his new best friends, James Cron and Conner Belle, to rescue the slaves. Can they?*

On the downside, Ben has hit puberty early and is aggressive and demanding on a constant basis with Alina. If he doesn't get what he wants, at times he even pushes or bites her. He only does this with Alina, and we are doing role-plays with the children to work on better options.

WEDNESDAY, OCTOBER 9, 2013

I gave Ben homemade bread made with amaranth flour and arrowroot this week. Donna Gates recommends flour every now and then on Body Ecology, if one can handle it. I don't think Ben can handle it. Today he laughed so hysterically at school he wet his pants. Then he was hysterical with giggles and circuiting tonight. Right now, at almost 9 PM, he is lying in his bed, muttering stories to himself. He is usually asleep by 8 or 8:30.

Finally, when I was tucking Ben in tonight, he asked me if I would hug him for a whole minute. He said, "I'll let you know when you can let go!" We hugged for a solid minute, both of us feeling our very special connection. Then he said, "Okay, you can let go now."

THURSDAY, OCTOBER 17, 2013

A note from Sean

"Something small seems monumental to me. Last night, Ben went with me to pick up Alina from her dance class so that they could tell each other a story on the way home. On the way there, I told Ben Alina might not want to do the story and that he should be prepared to be flexible. He said he would. Sure enough, Alina, tired as she was at that time of day, had no interest in doing the story. She just wanted to listen to music. Ben was disappointed, but dealt with it very well. Then, out of the blue, Alina rewarded Ben for coming with me to pick her up by promising him that as soon as she woke up, she would go into his room, and they could tell a story. Ben was elated.

"Then this morning, I heard Ben yelling. Not out of control, but clearly frustrated. I let them have their process without interfering and found them a few minutes later. Ben was playing with his toys, and Alina was reading a book. I sat down next to Alina and reminded her of last night's promise. She said she had remembered and went into his room this morning only to say that she needed some time before she would agree to share a story. She understood that is not what she had promised him, but she just didn't want to do it then.

"For Ben, stories help him find a way to channel all the thoughts and images in his head out of him in a controlled, enjoyable manner. They are therapeutic for him. So, when Alina came in this morning, Ben expected a story, and it was snatched away. I felt bad for Ben. I sat down next to him and told him that the hardest part of his life is his inability to control others, that he can't make other people do what he wants, and that I felt bad that Alina had made a promise and then changed it.

"Here is the amazing part. He turned to me and said, 'Thank you,' full of understanding and appreciation. In the past, Ben might have said, 'Go away,' or 'do we have to talk about this now?' or something like that. Or sometimes he might tell me to make Alina do the story, or he would try to bribe her (he likes to offer her food or give her money) or demand I punish her. But he simply said 'Thank you.'

Then, when I asked him if he would like to make his bed with me now or later (he needs a little help), he said now, in case he was in the middle of a story with Alina later.

"There was no sulking, anger, or any other reaction. He accepted, after a few minutes of frustration, Alina changing plans, and then, when I expressed empathy, he accepted it graciously and gratefully. The fact that I am writing so much about two words may seem silly to some, but it truly was an amazing moment."

SUNDAY, OCTOBER 27, 2013

At dinner last week, I served the children a new cauliflower dish. Ben looked at it, then looked at me incredulously. "Really, Mom? This is *cauliflower!*" "Ben," I implored, "just two bites. That's all." He tried a bite and grimaced. He looked up at me, disbelieving. "Oh Ben, don't be such a drama queen. Please, just two more bites?" Ben paused and looked at the vegetable on his plate. "Okay, I'll do it for *you*." He paused a second time, looked up directly into my eyes, and exclaimed, "But don't get used to it!"

FRIDAY, NOVEMBER 1, 2013

Ben has been pushing Alina physically a lot lately when she won't do what he asks. Tonight when we were reading *Harry Potter*, she refused to move so that Ben could have a turn sitting next to me. Ben got angry and pushed her in the chest, which is typically where he's been pushing her lately, sometimes quite hard. A fight ensued, with crying and drama. It lasted about fifteen minutes. I told Ben that I really, really wanted him to stop bullying and pushing Alina. It wasn't right, and it wasn't fair to me, because I had to then mediate between them. He listened but did not seem to take it in.

Later, as I was tucking him in, Ben shared some thoughts about himself. I started the conversation by saying that tomorrow was an exciting day, his last day as a ten-year-old.

Ben: Perhaps I shouldn't have my birthday, because I keep pushing Alina around.

Me: What, Ben? Do you mean you should be punished for that behavior? That seems strong, to lose your birthday!

Ben: When I'm pushing her, I'm more like a *six*-year-old, not an eleven-year-old.

Me: Well, sweetheart, we get stronger as we get older, and now that you will be eleven, you will be able to do better with Alina!

He grinned.

At *kiddush* tonight, as with many *kiddushes* lately, Ben's prayer for strength in the coming week was to fight less with Alina and the other kids at school. He wants to be a good person. Often, when he acts badly, bullying Alina, defying me, or refusing to do something he should be doing, he subsequently shows tremendous remorse, saying "I'm sorry I acted badly, I don't know what came over me," or "I don't know why I acted that way." I hope he will balance out, over time, so that he is able to be more in control of his feelings and actions.

SATURDAY, NOVEMBER 2, 2013

Tomorrow is Ben's birthday. When I asked him what he wanted to do for his birthday, he replied, "I just want to go out to dinner with my family." So that's what we're doing.

MONDAY, NOVEMBER 4, 2013

The other morning, Ben and Alina fought. Sean was watching the children while I took some quiet time. Ben ended up biting Alina, and all of this before 6 AM! When I came out, I went into Ben's room and spoke to him about what had happened. I asked him if he wanted to discuss it, and he replied, "Not really." So I decided to just be reassuring, since the incident was over by that point, and snuggled with Ben for a few moments. Sean entered the room a few minutes later, in order to help Ben make his bed.

Ben: [whispering] Sorry, Mom!

Me: It's okay, honey.

Sean: Why's Ben apologizing?

Me: Because he misbehaved earlier.

Ben: No, that's not why!

Me: Oh! Then why?

Ben: Because Dad interrupted our love meeting!

Wow. My son and I now have *love meetings.*

Don't be jealous. Maybe someday you'll get to have a love meeting, too.

SUNDAY, NOVEMBER 10, 2013

Yesterday Ben was working on Volume Two, Chapter Ten of his *Gabriel Garnet* series. Unfortunately, he lost a chunk of text and went into a state of total hysteria. He begged me to fix it. I did my best, but the text was lost. He proceeded to get very upset and threatened Alina, until Sean put Ben in his room to cool off.

Two minutes after being put in his bedroom, Ben pushed a piece of paper under the door and into the hallway. It read, "Dear Alina, I hope you write a book on the computer and its words vanish from the screen and it makes you cry. Ben." Alina, who was, in fact, busily working away on *her* book, *Samycake*, about three friends who go on adventures together, thought Ben's note was very funny. She responded, writing on Ben's paper, "I am working on Samycake!" She slipped the note under Ben's door. A minute later, the following note was pushed out: "Have any words disappeared yet?" Alina wrote back, "No, silly!" Ben quickly wrote back, "Well if you never do, you have to do my chores every day!" Alina responded, "Says who?"

After this, the children went back and forth, scribbling notes to one another, as follows:

Ben: Says the world. Everyone at school says that when a person makes a writing mistake another has to [make one] too, so the first person doesn't look like an idiot.

Alina: You do not look like an idiot. The world, also, doesn't say that.

Ben: Don't you understand my upset feeling?

Alina: I said you *don't* look like an idiot, not that you *do* look like one.

Ben: But I made a terrible embarrassing mistake on the computer. I mean I lost something and might never have it back.

Alina: I will help you write it! [smiley face]

Ben: Oh will you? Thank you. I'm so sorry.

Ben ultimately rewrote the chapter himself, with Alina looking on. I was one proud mama; talk about the pen conquering the sword! Sean and I marveled as we watched our son work through his feelings of frustration and embarrassment, and ultimately let go of those feelings through dialogue and communication with his sister. We *kvelled* as we observed our daughter's wit, diplomacy, and compassion for her big brother, despite their constant sibling-war dynamics.

MONDAY, NOVEMBER 11, 2013

Ben and I were alone this evening. Sean's in Boston, and Alina was asleep. We sat at the dining room table, so he could eat his night snack. As he ate, we chatted about things. We had spoken earlier in the day about IVIG and how much he hated it. I told him that I knew IVIG was lousy but that it was worth it if it helped him get better. Also, I said, because of the progress he's made through all the things that we have tried, he was already a source of great hope for parents with children who had autism. I explained that most parents are told, and believe, that if your child has autism, he or she can never get over it, and that Ben was an example of how much progress some kids actually can make if they get help.

As he ate, we continued the conversation. I told him there was a long period of time when I couldn't reach him, because of his autism, and that I was happy now to be able to just sit and talk to him. He said he remembered that period of time, when he didn't notice us "so much." He told me, amazingly, his version of an episode when he was around six (he remembered his age), when he ran out into the woods behind our home. Sean and I were terrified, and we called the police. By the time they arrived, Sean had tracked him down. The police at that time recommended an ankle GPS, which we declined. It was one of a series of horrible incidents where Ben ran away, and I went insane with fear.

Ben's version of that particular incident, as he revealed to me this evening, was quite different. He told me he had actually wanted to run a race with Daddy, but Daddy wasn't home. He knew that he knew his way around the woods, so he decided to race against imaginary people. He remembered we got upset and that the police came. But he had just wanted to run a race with Daddy.

I told him I didn't realize he was even aware of us at that time, much less wanting to run races with Daddy. He said he wasn't always. "My head," he told me, "was always full of the stories." He said this a little sadly.

"That's why I want you to keep doing IVIG even though it's so hard, sweetheart." Ben nodded.

I was shocked to hear that Ben was aware of us at that time to such an extent, despite outward appearances.

I think Ben has always been aware of others, and perhaps always desired to connect with others, but just didn't have the tools to do so. And he's up against the stories, stories that fill his mind and keep him from being present to what's happening outside his head and the world around him.

With Alina, it's different. If I invest myself in her, she gives me everything. Ben is constantly elusive and so complex. Alina is also not simple; she is just more easily reachable.

FRIDAY, NOVEMBER 15, 2013

I love the spontaneity of my conversations with Ben these days. Tonight, while he was writing and I was reading, Ben suddenly exclaimed, "Mom! Do you remember when I used to think there were only four sports? Basketball, baseball, soccer, and football." "Wow, Ben," I replied. "I didn't know that! But now you know there are others?" "Yeah. Hockey, tennis, lots." "What's your favorite sport these days?" "I don't really have a favorite right now." "I see." Then we went back to writing and reading.

MONDAY, NOVEMBER 18, 2013

I got a call from Ben's teacher today, who informed me that Ben has been showing extremely aberrant behavior for a week or so. Ben has apparently been:

- mean to the girls in his class (there are three girls; he is the only boy), especially to T., who has previously been his protector and ally. T. is extremely sensitive and has apparently felt Ben's meanness keenly;
- kissing the girls in his class, without their permission;
- talking about inappropriate things with the other children; and,
- more aggressive overall.

The teacher was quite concerned and remarked, "It's as though there is a Ben here we have never met before." I told her I would speak with him, and we would address these issues with our Son-Rise Program. She also asked about Ben's next IVIG treatment, commenting that she and the assistant teacher both saw more consciousness and being present after his last IVIG, both of which now seem to have faded. I explained to her that we have had two appointments canceled by the clinic, which means that Ben has not had IVIG for two months. I have been fighting to get a treatment this month, and I think I may have resolved the matter by finding a local provider.

I spoke with Ben about the teacher's call, and Ben wrote a letter to her, in which he took responsibility and apologized for his behavior. He promised in the letter to try to change, not talk about inappropriate things, and be kind. He wrote that if he breaks his promise he will eat twelve eggs—his most-hated food! He took it seriously, but he told me he is doubtful he will have the self-control to stop. He asked me to ask his teacher to call me tomorrow if he makes any mistakes, so that "you and I can work on these problems at home, Mommy!" I think he would rather stay home and work on them tomorrow, but I am not prepared, and I think he can do better than he thinks he can.

SUNDAY, NOVEMBER 24, 2013

Ben's behavior continues to worsen. He is aggressive, rigid, obsessive, demanding, and, at times, very nonresponsive. Sean and I chalk it up to puberty and the two-month gap in Ben's IVIG treatments, as a result of scheduling problems at the clinic. We are hopeful that eventual resumption of his monthly IVIG treatments will alleviate Ben's obsession and rigidity. But I am confused and a bit scared. The interventions we are currently using for Ben are as follows:

- Body Ecology Diet (sort of; I haven't added in the coconut kefir or the smoothies, which are a huge part of the Diet, or all of the supplements yet, but we are on our way);
- IVIG (monthly, assuming all continues to go well with insurance);
- the iMRS mat, which is supposed to be supplying Ben's cells with pulsed-electromagnetic fields to oxygenate and heal cellular degradation—or something like that;
- Heilkunst homeopathy to heal "shocks and traumas" to his "energetic body" (sounds like snake oil but has helped many, many children);
- exercise (Ben bikes and walks to school every day, and twice a week, we do soccer drills in the backyard with friends);
- executive skill work, with getting-ready-for-bed and getting-ready-for-school checklists I created and both children use;
- vision therapy, although that has not started as of yet; and,
- The Son-Rise Program, but only in our attitudes, not with actual, hands-on therapy anymore. And our Son-Rise Program attitudes slip constantly.

Ben is at times so "healed" that it appears he no longer meets an autism diagnosis. At other times, he becomes so rigid, demanding, nonresponsive, or obsessed that he seems in desperate need for something I am not providing.

So I wonder:

Should I be doing more? Is that even possible?

More to the point, is what we are doing having a substantial and meaningful effect?

Where is *my* textbook?

Where is *my* teacher?

I had lunch with a woman with a child on the spectrum last week, who is doing the CD-parasite protocol. We stopped CD last year, because the medicine we added, which was outside the main protocol, made Ben autistic. After he recovered from the medicine, I was too physically and mentally exhausted to continue with the CD, the required supplements, and the enemas. After chatting with her, I wondered, "Should we go back to *that* protocol? Is *that* where Ben's healing lies?" There is no roadmap to be found—anywhere or from anyone. Every child is different.

Every child has different needs at different times. Ben in puberty is different from Ben before puberty. He is more difficult in many ways, but he is also more awake, alive, funny, prolific, and interactive.

It's tough.

I feel so inadequate!

I've been beating myself up a lot lately. "If I were more organized . . ." "If I were smarter . . ." "If I were better at keeping records . . ." "Why didn't I remember to order that darn supplement last week? And now we've run out!" "Why can't I make that food turn out right?" "Why don't I know what to add when, or what's *really* working?" "Why can't I figure all this out? What if I fail him? What then? Where will he end up? Where will *we* end up? With what burden will Alina be left?"

I realized this week, yet again, that I am exhausted and not taking care of myself. If I'm going to stay this course, I have to put myself first with more consistency. I'm burning out physically, spiritually, and mentally, and it's taking its toll on my marriage and my parenting. If I don't feel good inside, I won't be able to help Ben heal. We will discover the answers to Ben's healing eventually. But I've gotten too tired. It's been one of those weeks.

Ben just called out to me, unsolicited, "Good night, Mom!"

I always forget: my *heart* is my textbook.

And Ben is my teacher.

THURSDAY, NOVEMBER 28, 2013

Tonight we had a wonderful Thanksgiving. We had at our table, among other friends and family, a family with a very impaired Son-Rise Program child named Ryan. At the end of the evening, my father remarked to Alina, "You were wonderful tonight with Ryan!" Without a moment's pause, Alina replied, "I've had a lot of experience."

WEDNESDAY, DECEMBER 4, 2013

A much better way to do IVIG!

Much has happened over the past several weeks. First of all, Ben had his sixth IVIG. For the first time, we did an at-home infusion, although "home" was a Marriott Hotel in Park Ridge, New Jersey, ten minutes from our actual home. We learned in November that we could do IVIG this way, and it was a much easier experience for Ben and all of us. Since his recent infusion, the rigid, explosive, physically aggressive, and demanding Ben has transformed once again into a gentle, much more flexible, less demanding, and happier Ben. Will it last? I'm taking it one infusion at a time for now.

We have found a temple community!

Then, Friday night at the temple, there was a Hanukkah Shabbat ceremony in which Ben's youth choir again sang. This time, they sang five songs, some with dancing! The joy on Ben's face was transcendent. He stayed with the group, he did the moves with the group, and you could just see how much a part of the group he felt. I felt like I was in someone else's life. After the temple choir sang, we sang the Hanukkah prayers and did the *kiddush*. Finally, our rabbi had each family light their menorah (everyone had brought menorahs from home). The menorahs were arranged on tables all around the sanctuary, and once they were all lit, the rabbi turned off the overhead lights. Our cantor played the guitar. The quiet room was lit with the light of many menorahs, glowing in colors in the darkness, and all of the families were holding each other in love and peace. The moment was wondrous.

We all sat together in a single pew: my parents, my children, my husband, our beloved au pair, Tim, who has become a true family member, and me. I thought of my brother and my grandmother, both of whom are gone, and felt them there with us. I felt the sacredness of family and community. We were there with each other, the congregation, and new friends, with whom we are spending time outside of temple and developing meaningful and delightful connections.

None of this was possible before Ben's recovery. Every experience we had prior to Ben's emergence, regardless of the beauty or meaning of that experience, was diminished by our awareness, as parents, that our son was unable to experience it with us. And there was always the disruptive behavior, and our expectations of that disruptive behavior, that compromised our ability to enjoy any public or shared experience with other families.

THURSDAY, DECEMBER 5, 2013

An email from Sean

Ben's growing up! This morning Ben suddenly brought up his little friend from Hebrew school and the fact that her family was over last night for the last night of Hanukkah. He said, "Last night I felt we were a C-O-U-P-L-E" spelling it out for me. My first thought was "how quaint a phrase!" and wondering where he found it, but I pushed those thoughts aside and said, "A couple." He nodded. I then said, "Do you have a crush on her?" He said no. I then suggested that a better description would then be BFFs. Ben replied, "I was thinking last night that we were a couple, it just felt like we were a couple." I asked, "Because you felt so close and comfortable with her?" He nodded yes. I celebrated the conversation and then had to go to work.

THURSDAY, DECEMBER 12, 2013

Last night I did a "liver flush," in which I drank a cup of Epsom salts and two hours later drank six ounces of olive oil. It was one of the most disgusting experiences of my life—truly terrible. I vomited partway through the oil, but eventually managed to get it all down. Today I feel horrid: nauseated and enervated.

Yesterday, when I told Ben that I needed to do this cleanse to get my liver healthy, he was so compassionate! He remarked, "Can I drink a smoothie or eat some eggs when you do this?" Ben *detests* eggs and smoothies. I was touched. This morning, I was lying in bed, feeling disgusting, and Ben came in. He asked me, "Can I snuggle with you?" I was thrilled, despite my nausea. "Sure, honey! Thanks!" So he got into bed with me and snuggled up close. After a few moments, Ben said, "I wish I was back before I was born, because then I could be with you all the time."

TUESDAY, DECEMBER 17, 2013

I was hard on Alina today. She eats too much, and I worry. I have my own past, self-destructive eating history, and I project my past experience onto her future.

I'm unfair; I am sharp with her at times, and I feel terrible about it.

Tonight, for example, she took a painting of Ben's from last year—one that I had never seen: a gorgeous painting of a rose within circles of color, it was really extraordinary, I didn't even know he could paint like that—and cut out pieces to use for a birthday card for her teacher. I was irate, and I cut her off at the knees. "*Alina! What are you doing with that?*" Alina literally jumped, startled, shock and fear registering in her whole body, especially her eyes. I apologized, but not before I said, "That's Ben's beautiful painting, how could you do that?" She just looked up at me and said, "I wanted it to make Mrs. Olson's card! I needed it." Afterward I felt terrible. I still do.

Then later she was eating a banana—her third fruit today—and I jumped down her throat. "You *know* what the doctor said about your back today!" I was referring to the fact that Alina's rather large tummy has pulled her back into a terrible curve, and either she has to do core-strengthening work in occupational therapy or she has to eat less. She opted for the therapy, but the point was clear that her belly is too big. I barked at her: "*Not another banana, Alina!*" Not good. I could alienate her. There has been so much tolerance of Ben's abnormalities and so much judgment of Alina's challenges. I don't identify with Ben's problems, and they seem so serious compared to Alina's. Ben's challenges frighten me, but they don't remind me of myself.

Parenting is confronting. It's a difficult gift. I never stop learning how to love. I want to learn from today. Control is not love.

FRIDAY, DECEMBER 20, 2013

Ben told me tonight he wanted to "have a chat to me" about something, and asked me if that would be okay. I was of course ecstatic. He then proceeded to share with me that other than his one little friend, he didn't feel that his Hebrew school friends were really "true friends" and not just acquaintances. I told him I agreed and that we should think of ways to deepen those connections.

I reminded him that boys usually like to talk about boyish things, and that perhaps he could talk to them about the fact that his favorite sport is basketball and that he just got a new bike from his grandparents. I also suggested we have a Shabbat dinner some week and do a potluck with some of the families. "It helps to spend time outside of the classroom," I suggested.

Finally, I told him how thrilled I was that he wants to develop these friendships and that if they do get to be friends, they will be lucky to have Ben as a friend. "Why?" Ben asked. "Because you are a really loyal and kind friend, Ben, and while you will be lucky to have new friends, they will be lucky to have that kind of friend in you." Ben grinned, "Even if I am blushing a little bit." Later we were snuggling while I was tucking him in, and he commented, after several sweet moments had gone silently by, "This is such a peaceful moment. Do you think we could let it last all night?" "Absolutely," I replied. He fell asleep soon after.

I feel sometimes—like tonight—as if God is making up for all those years of autism and disconnection by blessing me with these conversations that are so unexpected, open, brave, and trusting on Ben's part, and so intensely meaningful to me. I also think *Ben knows* how much it means to me that he shares these innermost feelings, desires, and fears of his with me. He's very intuitive and reads me like a book—probably always has—and I think part of his willingness to share such things is that he knows how happy I am when he does. When Ben reaches out to me, unsolicited, about issues in his life like these Hebrew-school friends, I feel my heart healing from old wounds. An acutely painful absence of connection with my son has been replaced by emotional intimacy and loving vulnerability—with an eleven-year-old!

EARLY JANUARY 2014

Ben met his angel last night . . . and told me about it

"When I was half asleep last night I heard someone singing to me 'Osay Shalom,' then I met that person, an angel named Molly. We had a conversation. I asked if her name was really Molly and if I could tell anyone about her. She said yes, but I wondered, 'Was it my imagination or had I really met an angel?' After talking to her I felt amazed. I told my parents and still wonder. I have a mystery."

THURSDAY, FEBRUARY 13, 2014

Three valentines from Ben to me—one day early.

Ben has to give a valentine to a classmate for their Secret Valentine party tomorrow. So tonight, in many different colors of colored pencils, he wrote this poem to his friend, Tanya:

Dear Tanya,
Happy Valentines Day.
Love's in the air, and in the trees.
Love is in the hearts of you and me.
Today love unlocks our hearts.
Today is as sweet as a fruit tart.
From your friend, Ben

When I later asked Ben where he had put his homework and his valentine for his friend, he responded, "On my finished-homework shelf, Mom!" I've been trying to get this kid to put his homework on his "finished-homework shelf" for six months with zero success. Why this sudden change tonight? No idea.

At dinner, for the first time in his life, Ben willingly ate fish. Chilean sea bass. At least two ounces. This is a major shift. In the past, Ben would no more have eaten fish than dirt. But tonight, he was fine with it. I asked him if he liked it, and he said, "Yes, but it's strange. Different." It's a textural thing; fish is different. But he was not revolted by it, which, given Ben's past reactions to new textures, maybe, is a sign of internal healing.

Afterwards, he even said he'd be willing to eat fish once or twice a week! The Body Ecology Diet seems to have balanced his blood pH and continues to heal his digestive system.

SUNDAY, FEBRUARY 16, 2014

Our first family-movie night

Tonight we watched *Diary of a Wimpy Kid*. Ben has never been willing to sit through an entire movie, even Harry Potter movies, even at home, because we are a Waldorf family. Ben knows movies are not part of Waldorf until children are older and has been rigid on this point. But both children love *Diary of a Wimpy Kid* books, and when we flew last week to Florida to visit Sean's parents, Alina watched the full-length movie, and Ben caught glimpses. Then last week, he asked me if we could get the movie to watch at home, and I was thrilled. I have always wanted to have a family-movie-night, despite my Waldorf soul. So today we went to the library, got the DVD, and watched it together this evening.

Ben's reaction was fascinating. Alina laughed the whole way through it. Ben, on the other hand, seemed entranced, in zombie mode, and I felt concerned. For the first hour, he just stared, expressionless, at the screen, laughing only once at one of the more slapstick moments. Otherwise, he seemed totally checked out.

Then at one point, some thuggy kids in the movie threatened to beat up Greg and Rowley, the movie's heroes. Ben exclaimed, "This movie is too violent!" Actually, it's about the least violent movie *ever*, next to *Teletubbies IV* or something like that. But Ben is very innocent, still, and didn't seem to know how to process threats against the movie's child heroes. After the movie was over, Ben continued, "Movies like that shouldn't be shown to kids our ages." I replied, "Mmm-hmm. Next time we'll find a more appropriate movie, honey." Ben was quick to caution me, "Not a baby movie, Mom. Just something more peaceful."

Peaceful but not babyish: I'm going to have to think about that, since every Disney or Pixar movie out there is filled with conflict, violence, and loss. Even the classics are rough!

Tonight I'm torn between feeling thrilled that Ben was willing to watch a movie and that we could have this kind of "normal-family experience," and on the other hand recognizing yet again that Ben still lives on a different plane and remains more sensitive, unblemished, pure, and undeveloped. I appreciate all of his sides. His is a remarkable process.

THURSDAY, MARCH 13, 2014

Ben got stuck tonight. He wanted his way; I don't even remember about what. He got frustrated, wouldn't listen, and shut down. And I couldn't let go. I couldn't see the big picture. I could only see him totally stuck, not progressing, all the past six years of work for nothing—he's still as stuck as he was—just a different focus. But still, still, stuck.

I cried, felt scared and sorry for myself, and let the feelings swallow me up. Sean guided me through it, without judging or trying to fix me. Eventually the emotional tidal wave subsided. In the meantime, Ben came into our bedroom and was desperate for me to feel better. "No one gets stuck the way I do! It's all my fault! I'm sorry, Mom! Is your nose red because you were crying?"

He put a piece of masking tape across his chest that read, "Mr. Meanie."

I'm carrying the world again, in my mind.

They're actually doing well, Ben and Alina. So he had an off day. Who doesn't?

Perspective. It eluded me tonight.

THURSDAY, MARCH 20, 2014

Things are different now

Tonight I was working in my home office on something with a deadline (a self-imposed deadline, but a deadline nonetheless), and Ben came in. He asked me to play with him, either to do a story or work on the movie he's currently writing. I responded instinctively, "I can't, Ben! I have to work!" He muttered, "Okay," and left the room.

Internally, I did a double take. I needed to work, I told my son I couldn't play with him, and off he went. Five years ago, even three years ago, Ben asking for me to play with him would have triggered an instantaneous *"Yes! Yes! Yes!"* from me. Because as recently as three to five years ago, Ben had little interest in looking at me, much less playing with me. But now Ben and I are so connected and interact so comfortably and frequently that I felt utterly within my rights to deny him my time today.

We started at total autism, with no desire for contact on his part and contact-*starvation* on my part. We moved next to consistent interaction but still with incredulity, inconsistency, and mistrust on my part. Today we have attained recovery—and I do mean *we*—on a level where I no longer feel desperate, needy, or terrified, but instead now fully expect that Ben will want me, love me, and want to spend time with me.

This journey is mine, as well as Ben's. I, too, have recovered so that I now trust his love. If I say no sometimes to Ben when he wants my time, I trust he will not subsequently reject me or go back to autism. A "normal" mother can't always give her child her time when there are other things that need to be done. Normal is not my standard, but trust in Ben's love— that has been my goal for a very, very long time. I'm getting there.

Remarkably, and notably, Ben's always been there.

SATURDAY, MARCH 22, 2014

When I was tucking Ben in this evening, Ben stroked my hair and remarked, looking into my eyes, "I hope you die before me. I just wouldn't want to be here without you."

MONDAY, MARCH 24, 2014

Note from Sean

"I learned that my father was in hospice this morning. Ben and Alina knew that he was sick and in the hospital, but they thought, because I thought, he was going to get better. Clearly that was not the case.

"Alina was home because she has a cold, and I told her the bad news. I planned to spend the morning with her and then go to work in the afternoon. I wanted to be there as much as possible after she knew her Zayde was going to die. I explained that he had been in pain for nine months, that his body wasn't getting better, and it was time for him to go. I explained that he had lived a wonderful life. I told to her what he had taught me: put family and work (in order to support the family) above everything. I told her Zayde had done just that. That his children had grown up and had families of their own and that he had worked until it was time to stop. That he had done everything he had set out to do and was ready to go. I told her I knew it wasn't fair, that she had only known him for nine years. I explained there was nothing to be done about it, but that it really was a blessing because he was out of pain. Alina cried some, but she also understood. We talked some and then resumed our activities.

"Later, she asked me to find out how her cousin Becca is doing because, 'We're basically the same person, and if I'm having a hard time with it, she is too.' So, when I found out Becca was sad, I let Alina know. I treated her like a young adult, and she responded beautifully.

"Ben was a completely different story. Not his behavior, but my expectations. I've been keeping the teachers updated with what's going on so they could be there to help the kids. I told Alina's teacher she knew and was doing okay with it. But I found myself writing to Ben's teacher that I didn't know what to expect, that I'd probably have to tell him twice. I read what I had written and was appalled. I deleted it and put the truth: that he didn't know and I would tell him tonight.

"So, tonight Ben was finishing dinner, and I sat down with him. I said, 'You know how Zayde is in the hospital?' He nodded yes. I continued, 'And you know how I said he was going to get better?' He nodded again. 'Well, he isn't going to get better.' I waited to let it sink in. He asked, 'You mean he's going to die?' I said yes. He asked, 'Is he dying of old age?' I thought about it and said that he was. Ben said that gave him some relief (the idea that he had lived his life). He asked how old he was, and I said 82. Ben said that's not as good as 100, or even 83. I said I understood, but we both agreed that he had lived a good life. Ben then commented that his dying was a sign of a change. I asked what kind of change, and he explained that he wouldn't have his Zayde anymore, I wouldn't have my father, and that Grandma Ro would be alone.

"Ben then said he wished he could stay eleven forever. I thought he meant as the rest of us age, and I teased him that I didn't want to keep paying for him to be in fourth grade forever. But he meant for the year to stretch out for all of us. That he didn't want this year, in which his first grandparent died, to end. I thought that was really beautiful. He then asked if he could mail Zayde a letter telling him how much he is going to miss him. I told him I thought that was a beautiful idea and that I was flying down on Thursday, and I could read it to him. He appreciated that.

"He then asked me if I felt the same way he was feeling when *my* grandfather died. I told him I was sad, like he was, but that his expression of his sorrow was much more poignant than how I expressed my feelings so many years before. It was also then that I realized Ben had looked at me the entire conversation. I celebrated him for looking at me.

"Ben's response was so heartfelt, sincere, and moving. It was beautiful."

TUESDAY, MARCH 25, 2014

Ben just asked me, "Hey Mom, did you put in the book about what happened at OT the other day?" "No, Ben, I forgot! Can you write it for me?" So Ben wrote:

"Alina came in to my OT session the other day, but I didn't want her there, so I asked her to leave, politely. Then a woman came in and commented that was a really nice way to explain. Most big brothers just pick on their little sisters. I admitted that I pick on her sometimes, and she said, 'Well I'm sure that you nicely asking her to leave would make up for it.' And Laura, my therapist, was like, 'Hey, that's a compliment!' The other woman was like, 'What?' Laura explained about how embarrassed I had been when she told me how handsome I was with my new haircut. I was like, 'Listen, looks when you talk about them are a little embarrassing. But if I had to be the best at anything, it would be to be the kindest person.' Laura was like, 'Whoa, most boys don't care about kindness and care about how they look. It's like you have your own—' I'm not sure what she said, your own personality or point of view or whatever. It's like I have my own cares or something."

Then he reminded me: "Make sure you put it in the book, Mom!"

WEDNESDAY, MARCH 26, 2014

*Another note from Sean, on Ben's goodbye conversation with Zayde,
who is currently unconscious and in hospice*

"I put Ben on speaker and explained that his Zayde would not be
able to speak to him, but he would hear Ben. Ben's first statement was
something to the effect of, 'Hi, Zayde. I really hate the fact you are
going to die. I'll miss you.' I then asked Ben if that is all he wanted to
say. He said to me, 'Dad, I'm confused. I love him and miss him.' I
replied, 'Then, Ben, that is what you should tell him.' I put him back
on speaker, and he said, 'I love you and miss you and I'm really sorry
I'll never hear your voice again.'

"I can't say for sure that Dad heard him, but his breathing did
intensify, so he may have heard Ben's voice. I choose to believe he did.

"Love you, Ben."

SUNDAY, APRIL 6, 2014

A new road for Mommy

I had a surprising experience today. I am studying to be a health-
and-nutrition coach for families of children with autism and other
immune-system-based disorders, and today I gave my first workshop on diet and integrative nutrition for those types of issues. I
presented to a small group of mothers, all with children with varying
special needs. I discussed the life-altering, yet inexpensive, uses of
Epsom salts, coconut oil, and apple cider vinegar. I discussed the
connection between alkalinity, acidity, and pathogenic bacteria in
the body. I discussed the critical importance of the gut in relation
to serotonin production, the immune system, and the second brain.
I presented demos of various brain-boosting, immune-enhancing,

and child-loving recipes, such as avocado-chocolate (cacao) pudding, buckwheat bread (with only two ingredients!), seed grains, sea vegetables, super-easy super-food cereal, and several other foods.

I'm doing this partly because after seven years of uninsured medical expenses and special diets for autism recovery, we need money. I'm also doing it because I love families and have always sought a way to help them, initially by becoming a family lawyer.

But this might be it. Although I had no inkling of the happiness I would feel after presenting to these mothers today, tonight I feel great, and I know it's because I gave these women a few tools to add to their arsenal against their children's challenges. I gave them some new ideas, some simple changes, and some inexpensive alternatives to what they have been doing, and these new things might actually make a difference for them and their kids. If I believe what I'm doing will help others—then I can throw everything I have into it. This might be it.

The coolest thing about today? The children at the workshop loved the foods we made!

FRIDAY, APRIL 11, 2014

Careful what you pray for

I think I liked it better when Ben was autistic.

It's just tonight he called me on my stuff. The children and I were having a relaxed, peaceful, and really fun evening reading. Sean was at temple, saying Kaddish for his father, who passed away two weeks ago.

Suddenly I realized the time and told the children it was time for bed. They muttered, "Uh-huh." I went into the kitchen to clean up a bit, and when I came back, neither child had moved an inch. I said, "Guys, it's time to stop reading. It's bedtime." Neither budged. "*Guys!*" I yelled, in a sudden rage, "*Come on! I am so sick of you not responding when I ask you to stop reading!*" Alina jumped up, said "Sorry, Mom," and went to get ready for bed.

Ben looked up at me, paused, and said, "Wow."

Wow?

At that moment, I saw a choice in front of me; namely, I could keep yelling or I could laugh at myself. Thankfully, I laughed.

Then I asked, "Why 'wow,' Ben?"

He replied, "Why do you have to be so moody?" He looked me right in the eyes.

Fair enough.

Not much I could say to that.

Like I said, I think I liked it better when he was autistic.

SATURDAY, APRIL 19, 2014

Funny memory tonight. Years ago, Ben never sat with us at holiday dinners. He sat separately, even in a separate room. Then a few years ago, several years into our Son-Rise Program, Ben spent an entire Thanksgiving dinner *underneath* the table. At the time, that was progress! I slid plates full of food under, and Ben slid empty plates out. The following year, Alina joined Ben under the table, and it was more playful and less autistic.

This year? We held a Seder at our home this evening, and it was beautiful. Sean gave a speech about his father. I designed a *haggadah* that we used, and we read from Dr. Martin Luther King, Jr., Anne Frank, and the poet, Anthony Hecht, among others. Ben read along with everything, even sang the Hebrew prayers when it came to his turn. He was exemplary, a perfectly behaved participant in the ceremony. Around eight o'clock, he got very tired—as did we all—and it was clear he was done for the evening. He said his proper goodbyes to our guests and went off to read in bed.

THURSDAY, MAY 29, 2014

Ben's movie

Ben is directing a movie about American Girl historical dolls and the respective societies in which they live. There are chapters at the end of each American Girl Doll book called "Looking Back," and Ben is turning those chapters—which describe the culture and politics of the respective eras—into monologues to be performed by each of the "dolls," who will in turn be played by various young actress friends of ours. Ben has decided to call the movie itself *Looking Back*, just like the chapters. He wants it to be an educational piece to be used in schools. It's a great innovation, as are many of Ben's ideas.

For many weeks, he has been dictating the "Looking Back" chapters from each of the books while I type. I type about eighty words per minute, so we fly through the chapters, and it's a lot of fun. I love working on this project with Ben. It's fun, smart, and a beautiful way to spend time together. Ben's selection of the various actresses to play the various doll-parts is also very charming. He wants the girls to somewhat resemble the parts they will portray in the movie.

Yesterday Ben went to a birthday party for his friend from Hebrew school, and spent time with another little girl who was also at the party. Today Ben asked me to ask this girl's mom if she would like to be in his movie, and her mother responded with a strong affirmative from Brooke. She also commented that this new little friend thinks Ben is really nice. Ben also met a boy at the party who is Ben's age. The two boys spent much of the party playing games and hanging out together, and Ben was very excited. Ben remarked to me, just now as we were finishing up another Looking Back chapter, "Mom, do you know what I'm realizing? The more things I do, like Hebrew school, and the party yesterday, the more friends I make!And I'm making a lot of friends!"

THURSDAY, JUNE 5, 2014

Tonight after prayers, I said, "And thank you God for *Benjamin*, whom I love so much," and Ben interjected, "And for *Susan!*" Then he added, "Was that weird that I called you Susan?" "Not at all, Ben, not at all," I replied.

***

Chapters 3 and 4, "Emergence" and "Struggling To Connect," presented the process through which Ben emerged from the cocoon of autism and began unfurling his wings. In Chapter 5, "Conversations and Connections," many of Ben's deepest desires were fulfilled, through the development of true, sustained friendships and participation with peers in healthy school and after-school environments. The two years since we moved to New York have unquestionably been fraught with emotional ups and downs, ongoing systemic, biomedical challenges, and serious social errors by Ben. Especially in the first year of the move, Ben continually went in and out of autistic behaviors, and I fought hard to sustain my hope and conviction that he would ultimately fully recover someday. Additionally, during that first year, Ben, at age ten, hit early puberty, which brought on periods of violent and erratic behavior. We obtained support and guidance from our Son-Rise Program teachers, but the challenges were great.

Yet for every downturn, we were rewarded for our patience with meaningful and exciting shifts upward. Ben now expresses himself—his feelings, observations, and experiences—with an ever-increasing clarity, perception, and humor. Due to his love of reading and his immense capacity for devouring books—everything from childish chapter books to Harry Potter, The Hardy Boys, and Lemony Snicket—Ben's vocabulary expanded to college level. He became able and eager to express himself, through both writing and speaking, and did so constantly and with great enthusiasm. His friendships improved because his ability to communicate improved.

We are by no means out of the woods yet with regards to Ben's immune-system problems and accordant behavioral problems. Ben is not "cured." Sean and I still intermittently experience bouts of anxiety and self-pity. But we are always able to help each other regain perspective and, ultimately, find our way to hope once again. We continue to pursue biomedical interventions, and we maintain a commitment to Son-Rise Program principles within our home, though with Ben in school and participating in after-school activities, he no longer spends time in his Son-Rise Program playroom. Ben has speech challenges, and we still deal with PANDAS symptoms such as OCD and bathroom phobias.

But through his experiences at Otto Specht, as well as the other social environments into which he has been welcomed since we moved (such as our new temple, which has become a spiritual home for Ben), Ben has developed self-confidence, awareness of the feelings and needs of others, and friendships with children his age. People often don't realize Ben still has autistic tendencies, and he is growing, improving, and progressing constantly. Unlike in previous years, we are now able to have "normal" family experiences, such as incident-free family vacations, attendance at family life-cycle events, summer camp, harmonious visits with his grandparents both in our home and theirs, other travel, and an abundance of playdates. We still believe in Ben's capacity for total recovery. He is well on his way.

PART III:

WE ALL HAVE SPECIAL NEEDS

Chapter 6
Family Relationships

*B*en's autism is a gift, because it taught me how to love. It taught me to see the beauty in every child. It healed me from my fear of special needs, instilled in me from my childhood with Danny.

I no longer believe I caused Ben's autism. Maybe it was the vaccines, maybe the home birth and the lack of oxygen for that first eight minutes before the paramedics arrived, maybe something resulting from the IVF treatments, maybe something in his genetics. We'll never know. But I no longer believe it was my fault.

I also spend much less time comparing our family to other families. I no longer believe that parents of neurotypical children have it any easier than I do. Sure, maybe their roads are different, their kids' diets don't have to be as restricted as Ben's does, their money doesn't have to be poured into biomedical testing that no insurance company in the country covers or into au pairs and paid Son-Rise Program staff.

But I don't think those parents experience more love or happiness than Sean and I do having Ben in our lives. Ben and Alina have a close and meaningful relationship, in spite of and maybe even partly because of Ben's autism. I pity myself less than I used to for having a child with special needs, because I am grateful that Ben is Ben. If he has autism, well, then, that's part of Ben and so be it. Similarly, Alina has a temper and a food problem, and that is Alina, but that is not all she is. Autism is not all of who Ben has been. After years of traveling along this healing journey, I am learning to love Ben for all of who he is, rather than focusing on who he is not. What a way to love. What a model for loving that I can bring into all of my relationships.

I understand now that all children have special needs. I believe this, having lived with Ben and Alina and having had the privilege of connecting with many other children, mostly non-autistic and without a special-needs label. Every parent faces her child's limitations, and every parent can choose to focus on that child's beauty and gifts. The Son-Rise Program taught me to do that with my children.

And it's not just the children! Based on my observations, all adults have special needs. We're all learning how to emerge from isolation, interact in healthy ways, be interested in others, and mediate our idiosyncrasies within a social community. It isn't easy for any of us, unless we are lucky enough to somehow discover that to be authentically ourselves is all that's required, that it's safe to let go of fear and control, and that it matters more what we think of ourselves than what others think of us.

Before we all changed, life with Ben was painful, scary, and lonely. For the past three and a half years, Sean and I have used the new principles we learned to discover our son, our daughter, and ourselves from a radical and liberating new perspective. Ben is now engaged and in relationships with other people. But it is not just Ben. We are all changing.

***

Autism leaves its mark not just on the child, but on every member of that child's family. While trying to help Ben, we learned how to take care of Alina, help our marriage, and most importantly, take care of ourselves as individuals. This chapter is devoted to all family members.

MARRIAGE

The divorce statistics on parents of children with autism are frightening. Although the often-quoted statistic that 80 percent of parents with children with autism divorce appears to be only an urban legend*, trauma of any type wields a brutal sword against marital harmony. Parenting a child with autism—with any special needs, in fact—is terribly traumatic. I was lucky, however, because I grew up with magnificent teachers: my parents.

My brother's untimely death devastated my parents for years. Ultimately, however, they were able to heal sufficiently to face life with appreciation for what remained: namely, their marriage, me, good work, and the beauty of life (through music, art, poetry, and relationships). They remain two of the happiest people I know. Despite their loss, they successfully retained their compassion, their engagement with life, and a genuine *joie de vivre*.

So when life handed *me* a parental trauma—autism—I had fantastic role models to turn to for inspiration. It's no coincidence that I ultimately decided to embrace life—including Ben, whose autism frightened me for years—and to retain *my* compassion, *my* engagement with life, and even my *joie de vivre*.

My parents also chose to embrace each other, rather than to let their loss destroy their marriage. Again, it is no coincidence that after almost twelve years of living with a child with autism, who still struggles with attention problems and other autistic tendencies, our marriage has never been stronger. How has this happened? My husband and I, through many courses, consultations, and long evenings talking things through, adopted certain practices, all of which transformed our marriage:
1. We look for the good in each other.

---

* See Alysia Abbot, "Love in the Time of Autism," last reviewed September 10, 2013, http://www.psychologytoday.com/articles/201306/love-in-the-time-autism.

2. When we communicate, we actually *listen* to each other.

3. We maintain a high level of transparency in our communication. We don't lie to each other (most of the time), and we come clean when we have made an error that affects the other.

4. We try to remember that timing is critical in relationships and wait to say something hard until the person is in a place to hear it.

5. When one of us is angry at the other, we try to walk in their shoes (figuratively speaking) before *blasting* them.

6. We try to give more of ourselves than is comfortable and, yet, take care of ourselves at the same time. Assessing whose need is greater in a given moment requires honesty with ourselves and then with each other.

Struggles with children can forge a unique bond in parents who are committed to loving themselves, each other, and their children. If parents can disagree, argue, and even wage war occasionally, and then let it all go and embrace each other, the marriage may struggle, but it won't crash and burn. If parents can learn to listen to one another and take care of each other without needing a quid pro quo (or even a thank you), then a child's autism can become a vehicle for developing a deeply loving relationship. Thankfully, this is our experience.

But don't expect it to be fun.
Our multitude of arguments, tongue-lashings, misunderstandings, and mistaken assumptions could fill a book, and the many moments in which I knew I was being unreasonable, but my ego wouldn't let me stop and acknowledge the invalidity of my point, could fill a sequel. But in the aggregate, we've grown. We've learned to separate ourselves from our ego-driven pettiness and humble ourselves

in the moment. We have learned to let go—much of the time—of needing to be right at the expense of our relationship. Finally, we've learned, in the words of Phyllis Diller, that it's actually better to go to bed angry sometimes than to stay up all night fighting!

A few of our choice moments follow below, all part of the "marriage education" my husband and I received and continue to receive through parenting a child with autism.

FRIDAY, AUGUST 26, 2011

Blog entry from Sean, "A Case Study in Differing Parenting Styles, Consequences: Yea or Nay?"

Susan and I had an interesting night tonight. It all concerns the word "consequences." It really comes from a philosophy, and I seriously have no idea which one of us, if either of us, is right. I believe in consequences. I am not sure if Susan does or doesn't believe in them, but she does seem to have a reluctance to follow through on them.

Tonight

It all started with Ben (of course). Susan and the children went to the library today and picked up about a dozen books. (A lot of them involved a superhero called "Captain Underpants!") Anyway, Ben has this problem—he really gets into his books. Truthfully, I can relate, as I also hate putting down a book once I start it. So, this evening, when it was dinnertime, we had to ask him to come to the table four or five times. Susan asked him the first few times. Then I bent down and told him what he was doing was rude. He heard me and, with some resistance, went to the table and ate his dinner. But it all began again when it was time for his night snack. Ben didn't want to put down his book. Again, after several requests, he sat down. But then he went right back to his book instead of coming upstairs.

Our normal routine

The thing is, we have a ritual. The kids are supposed to go to bed no later than 8, but really closer to 7:30. Before he goes to bed, Ben comes upstairs, where I apply several different kinds of cream. Then I read to him while he drinks water with some supplements; then we brush his teeth and have prayers and singing.

My approach

So, tonight, I was upstairs getting their rooms ready for them to go to bed while Susan was trying to cajole Ben to go upstairs. I didn't fully hear what Susan was saying, but I believe, in essence, she was trying to explain to Ben that he can't be acting this way, especially when he is in WiSH school; if the teacher asks him to do something, he needs to do it. I could hear the frustration in her voice, so I went downstairs and inserted myself. (Yes, without consulting or talking to Susan).

I said to Susan that it's okay, Ben would just have the consequences of not taking part in his usual routine of reading or prayers and singing. Susan then responded that he must always do prayers, so I said fine, we'd just not do the reading. Susan hoped Ben would hear what she was saying. I didn't think he would, and I asked him later. During this whole process, Ben stayed glued to his book—I don't think he heard a thing either of us said. (Not that it bothered me, this is part of Ben, something we want to help him change, but I chose to stay happy about it).

Ben's reaction

So then Ben ran up to his room and shut his door. I followed him up, and I saw him peeping his head out the door with this sheepish grin on his face. I took my cue from his face. The first thing I did was let him know I wasn't angry or upset with him. I then asked him to take off his clothes, so we could start getting ready for bed.

While he was taking off his clothes, I began to explain to him about consequences. I started by asking him what happened if someone eats too much. He answered that you get an upset stomach. I told him he was right. Then I asked him what time it was. He said 8:02. And I said, "You're supposed to go to sleep by 8, right?" He said yes. I then reminded him of the things that had occurred that made it so late, including his being late to dinner, night snack, and coming upstairs. I further explained that the consequence of his being so late was that we wouldn't be reading to him.

Ben became upset. But significantly, Ben continued to get ready for bed. In past times, Ben would get upset and lose control, maybe go after Alina or just scream or whatever. But he let me put his cream on him and put on his pajamas. Then with a little encouragement, he drank his water. I thought it was great that he was staying with me despite being upset. I kept talking to him. Ben then began coming up with unique ways to resolve the situation.

The contrast with Alina is amazing. If I had explained to Alina what had happened and the consequence of the action, she would have apologized. She might have tried to get me to read a story, but she would have gotten it.

With Ben, he first suggested skipping prayers and singing instead. I laughed inside because I had suggested that earlier to Susan, but she had said no, prayers are not optional. So I explained to Ben that prayers are required just like brushing his teeth.

Then Ben suggested he clone me. He got a little rough with me and pulled my hair a few times. I stayed happy and loving. I told him it was fine if he cloned me; my clone would notice the time and ask him why he was still awake. It went on like this for twenty minutes. But what was great during this time was that Ben remained compliant. He got into bed.

Then something odd occurred. He began to want to punish us, also. For example, he kept trying to focus on Alina, wanting her to do something wrong so that she could have a consequence. I kept telling him that we were focusing on him, not her. Then he began wanting to punish us by having us sleep on the floor. I explained that would hurt Mommy's back. He got that.

Susan's approach

I was only in the room alone with Ben for, say, twenty minutes. Then Susan was up there for another fifteen minutes. She wanted Ben to understand why his action wasn't proper and that if he acted that way in school, his actions wouldn't be accepted. Susan tried to help Ben understand the situation. She went so far as to suggest to him that if he acknowledged the circumstances, I'd read to him. She promised him that if he said he understood and promised to be more compliant in the future, then I would read to him.

I protested, in part because I believed that his having experienced a taste of consequences was not enough and that we'd be rewarding his crying. Susan explained her distinction was that we were rewarding his understanding. Ben chose not to accept her offer anyway and still kept trying to come up with unique ways to resolve the situation.

My feelings about the experience

By 8:30, he had gone to bed, and we left the room. I felt great. I was thrilled that throughout the process Ben never checked out or freaked out. He had gotten upset but never stopped communicating with us.

We talked. Susan said she felt using the word consequences was threatening a result. I explained I felt otherwise. I think of consequences as a natural reaction to what has already occurred. You stay up late, the next day you are tired. You read too late, you don't get your bedtime story. I can't say for sure that Ben understood the circumstances. I'm not sure it will be different next time. I was okay with that. Susan was worried, because she thinks she might be scaring Ben about school. I told her I thought she did fine, that she built upon her conversations with Ben and kept communicating with him. She wasn't so sure.

Bottom lines

I know Susan and I should have talked more, set a plan, and so forth, but how can you plan for this stuff? If Ben is going to a school, we need to try to treat him like a normal child but still be flexible to understand Ben is not yet a normal child. Most importantly, we need to stay happy while doing it.

So here is my question—can you give a child still on the spectrum consequences?

My response to Sean's question (from Susan)

At Stage 4, we do need to give Ben consequences. Sean was right; I was afraid to follow through on the consequences last night. In the cool, unemotional light of dawn, I see that clearly. Especially given Ben's comments this morning that, "I don't want to miss stories tonight, so I'm going to listen when it's time to come to the table." Wow. The effectiveness of Sean's approach blew me away.

We are all learning and growing. I have a lot to learn from Sean about trusting Ben and not being afraid to set firm boundaries. Sean and I had different upbringings, and in some ways, Sean's parents did a better job with discipline. I'm grateful Sean and I can balance each other out and learn and grow together. I'm not always enjoying the process, but I'm thrilled with the results. Not just in Ben, but in the ever-growing, mutual respect and loving teamwork between Sean and me.

And God help me to keep my sense of humor!

FRIDAY, JANUARY 13, 2012

Sean and I are on a staycation for five days, at a Marriott about forty minutes from home. Tonight we went out to dinner at Longhorn Steakhouse. I had trout; Sean had steak tips. We talked about our marriage, loving each other more now than ever, and judging each other less and accepting, cherishing, and appreciating each other more as we grow older. We agreed that we need to talk about these things more, and that we may or may not talk about these things more, but that we were grateful for our time right now.

Then we went back to the hotel, and the children called to do prayers. I talked to both kids. Alina was affectionate, and Ben was extremely responsive. Sean got on the phone and talked to them.

JULY 2014

A typical stupid argument (on our way home from the Berkshires)

Sean: So what supplements are you giving Ben now? I thought you had started the B12 shots.

Susan: Why are you asking me that? I told you I had to go low and slow, one new supplement every three days. Didn't you see the pouches I made up for the trip? They have a lot of new ones in there.

Sean: Yes, I was confused because you said we were starting the shots right after the allergy-serum nose spray.

Susan: I did not say that. I said I was going through the supplements, one by one, three days apart. [Internally: *Did I say I would do the shots next? Darn it!*]

Sean: Fine, I just didn't understand.

Susan: Well, you sound very critical of me. I'm doing the best I can.

Sean: I know you are. As I said, I just didn't understand. Are you going to start the shots now?

Susan: I don't know. I don't know if that makes sense. I mean we're moving next week. [Internally: God, should I start the shots this week? Should I not have waited? Why did I wait? Darn it!]

Sean: What does moving have to do with the shots?

Susan: It just seems like a lot. Ben's going to have a fit when he hears he has to take shots twice a week. [*I don't think I can face giving him shots again.*]

Sean: It's up to you. I just want to make sure we're staying on track.

Susan: What do you mean by that? We are doing fine! We still have four or five supplements to add in. Sean, you are being so critical! Jesus! [*Am I screwing this up? I thought I was on top of this! Darn it!*]

Sean: You're overreacting.

Susan: [*I know I am. I'm embarrassed. I doubt myself.*] I am not. You're being unfair. I have to handle so much. I thought I did a great job getting everything ready.

Sean: You did.

Susan: So why are you being so hard on me?

On and on and on. I know what is happening in me, but I lash out because I am afraid I am failing Ben. Failing him again. Will I never forgive myself?

There is no arrival point.

SIBLINGS

Being the sibling of a child with autism is extremely complicated.

Growing up with a physically disabled older brother, I had very mixed feelings. I felt self-conscious at times. Why did he have to be so awkward and tell stupid jokes? Why did he have to try too hard and make everyone uncomfortable? Why couldn't he just relax? I felt embarrassed.

But as self-conscious as I felt at times, Danny was still my brother, whom I loved more than anybody except my parents. Danny and I had a special world, in which we experienced a sense of total familiarity and safety. I knew Danny thought I was great, and he knew I loved him just as much.

I also admired him. Danny was great at writing and building model planes and submarines. He understood a little about politics. He was patient and sang well. He was funny and made me laugh. He also knew things about me nobody else knew—like when I stole money from my parents for food—but he never told anyone, including my parents: he was loyal. He loved me more than anything.

My feelings about Danny were complicated. When bullies picked on him, I was heartsick and furious. But I judged him, and I wanted him to be normal. As a child, I didn't think so much about these things, but as an adult, I can see the internal confusion I struggled with. Today, I see the same ambivalence in Alina. At camp last summer, for example, she went through an uncomfortable time, in which she feared other children would identify *her* with Ben's disability.

THURSDAY, JUNE 27, 2013

Alina told me this morning that some kids in her bunk think Ben is weird. I asked her how she felt about that, and she said, "Bad, because he's my brother, and we're family so it's like they think I'm weird too." I didn't know what to say. I told her about some similar experiences I had as a child with Danny, but she lost interest in the conversation. I reiterated later that Ben is still "weird" to some people who only see his outward behavior and don't know how amazing, loving, funny, and smart he is inside. I said he's gotten better and will continue to get better. Finally, I reminded her that he is separate from her.

I wanted to give her better words, but I know the important thing is that she had someone to speak to and that she chose to talk to me about it.

***

Part of being the sibling of a child with special needs is the guilt the sibling feels for *having* mixed feelings. It feels disloyal to judge your brother or sister with disabilities. But a child desires connection with others more than anything, and challenges like autism separate a child from those others whose acceptance feels paramount. Accordingly, autistic behaviors inspire fear in the sibling, and that fear can easily morph into judgment. Judgment causes guilt, and the psychological vicious cycle is complete. This analysis may not fit every sibling of a child with special needs, but it was true for me.

Alina also expressed, more than once, her fear that we favored Ben over her, and her concern was valid. In our eagerness to please Ben, who had previously never given either of us the time of day, Sean and I indulged in a constant double standard when it came to the children. Up to a certain point, we rarely, if ever, said no to Ben when he

UNLOCKED

wanted something, even something unreasonable. Yet we often denied Alina's requests, which was appropriate, but in contrast to our permissiveness with Ben, appeared completely inequitable.

Underlying this double standard was the fact that I knew Alina would not retreat into autism even if I denied her requests, whereas the same was not true for Ben. Alina, supremely perceptive, felt the contrast keenly, as she shared with us at certain times.

In addition to this double standard, Alina also got the short end of the parenting stick all too often, when I felt depleted after going through a bad situation with Ben, and I had nothing left to offer to Alina in regards to energy, creativity, or enthusiasm.

FRIDAY, APRIL 5, 2013

I had a game planned, which I have been working on all week and which I completed this afternoon in anticipation of playing it with both children after school. The game is fabulous, a really great Son-Rise Program game, filled with Ben's motivators and hidden social challenges. We were all about to play the game, Ben, Alina, and I, when Ben got stuck, and I responded by getting stuck myself. Alina, immensely frustrated and disappointed, left the room. Once again, Ben spoiled it for her, for all of us, and I enabled it to happen. Instead of letting Ben have his temper tantrum and us play the game without him, I focused on Ben and ignored Alina's needs. Because I wanted Ben to let go, and not be stuck, to not be autistic. Once again, I responded with anger, impatience, and intolerance.

Later, I let Ben go back on the computer, and he resolved his issue. In other words, I caved. I showed him that unhappiness will get him what he wants. Then I was "a genius, the best mother in the world, etc." Ben was contrite the rest of the day, gracious, accommodating, and responsive to my questions. I'm trying not to be hard on myself,

310

but I didn't handle it well. I picked up fear, anger, and rigidity, and I will do it differently next time. I can let him be unhappy, if that's what he chooses. I can trust in his ability to find his way out of it without me giving him what he wants if it's not good for him. I can stay happy myself, resist the urge to be impatient, and most important, ask God to help me trust that Ben will be okay even if he decides to choose unhappiness for a while.

I can pay attention to Alina. I can put Ben in God's hands.

SUNDAY, APRIL 7, 2013

Alina wound up just playing by herself. I was worried she felt discounted, and it turns out I was right. She had wanted to play a new Son-Rise Program game I had created for us all to play together, and because Ben got rigid and nasty and I couldn't just let go and let him deal with his unhappiness. Alina has a bad habit of being rude to me at meals. Specifically, when I bring her meal out, she is critical and can be insulting. She was rude to me this afternoon about her snack, for example. I told her that was fine, but I didn't have to give her a snack she didn't want, and took it away. She burst into tears. I told her she could cry as long as she needed to, but I would prefer she do it in her room. She cries a lot to get her way, and we, unfortunately, have given in so many times that she has learned it is a good tool.

Anyway, she slammed her door a few times in a row and actually broke it. When I saw what she had done, I called Sean, and he was able to fix it, but not before we showed Alina what she had done. She became very remorseful and cried even more, saying, "I'm terrible!" a few times.

After the dust settled, I sat down and celebrated her for being a wonderful person. She said, "I don't feel that way." I replied, "Well, you acted badly this afternoon, but you can learn from it. I want you

311

to be appreciative and respectful of Daddy and me, and not rude. You can work on that and get better. You're a wonderful person; we just want you to be all you can be."

Alina nodded, and then she said, "I feel like Ben is more important. You pay more attention to him. I feel neglected." Where did she hear that word, I wondered. She continued, "I want to play with you a lot lately, but you're too busy doing stories with Ben." I am grateful for an open dialogue with both of my children. I have an opportunity to do better with both of them. Each day is a new beginning, with new moments to create. Just like Alina, I can do better. And I plan to.

***

Despite complicated feelings on Alina's part, she has been essential to Ben's recovery. She has taught him *more than anyone else* about connection, as well as about the rules of children's social interaction. She has not treated him as a special-needs child, but rather as her big brother whom she loves and drives crazy by turns.

Alina has also benefited from having Ben in her life. Ben and Alina share a language of story telling, which for him is the hallmark of his autism/OCD, but for her is merely joyful and creative play with her brother. They have spent literally hundreds of hours telling extemporaneous stories and reading together, bonding in a most intimate friendship, even before Ben had the skills to bond with anyone else. In Alina's eyes, Ben has never been *inadequate*; he is her brother. They share a pure sibling love that enhances and nourishes both of them, despite Ben's challenges. Ben feels about Alina the way Danny felt about me: she is utterly essential to his happiness, and she absolutely knows it. Given her own set of insecurities, for Alina to have a brother who worships her is not a bad thing. Overall, Alina is, today, a bright, happy, and thriving child, and there is no doubt that her relationship with Ben has been a critical factor in her development.

As a mother, I have "never enough" syndrome, as a result of which I judge myself too harshly and at times lose perspective regarding Alina, who has had a wonderful life despite our situation. Nevertheless, I have made great efforts to nurture her. Most importantly, I have given her my time and attention. I have consistently and tangibly invested myself in her, totally separate from my time with Ben or with the two of them. We take "Mommy and Alina days," where we go to dinner, a movie, or even a hotel—just the two of us. We do crafts together, just the two of us. We do "Ladies' Luncheons" with the grandmothers; no boys allowed!

I am also consistent with certain rituals we have developed together over the years of her childhood. I kiss her good night *every night*, for example, and do our special just-us prayers. I show her I trust and believe in her by letting her help me prepare meals or pick out my outfits for parties. I frequently ask her how she is feeling about the different areas of her life, and I listen carefully to her answers.

Finally, I now say no to Ben sometimes. I treat the children as similarly and as fairly as I can.

All of these actions—done imperfectly, as always—have added up to a remarkably secure child, despite our immense focus on Ben's autism and recovery.

SUNDAY, JANUARY 1, 2012

Then there's Alina. Endlessly brilliant, beautiful, stylish, creative, imaginative, loving, adoring, and so adorable it ought to be illegal. She gets more special to me every day. No particular moment on which to report—just an ongoing, heartfelt gratitude for who she is and that I get to be her one and only Mommy.

SUNDAY, FEBRUARY 10, 2012

Our darling Alina lost her first tooth this evening. I actually pulled it out, because it's been loose for weeks. She is thrilled, and the "lamb fairy" will be paying her a lucrative visit this night! (For Ben it was the pig fairy; our little girl would like a lamb.) I feel blessed to share in these moments with our children.

TUESDAY, JULY 15, 2014

"Ninety pounds???????? Ninety pounds???????"

I entered our bedroom, to see my nine-year-old daughter slumped on our bed, head in her hands. She looked up at me, huge blue eyes brimming. "Mom? Ninety pounds? Mom?"

I got her point instantly: my beautiful, talented, precocious, kind-hearted daughter, Alina, has a food and weight problem—just like her dear ol' mom. Only I discovered a way out when I was twenty and haven't struggled since. Alina, on the other hand, is in the throes of cravings and food obsessions that bother her constantly, especially since they lead to overeating and a chubby physique.

I lay down on the bed with her and tried to offer words of comfort. Tonight, I think, I actually got it right: I validated her, empathized with her, and gave her a sense of control. At least it seemed so. The backstory is that Alina also weighed herself just yesterday morning, and weighed eighty-nine pounds. I need to put away the scale.

Alina: Ninety pounds, Mom?

Mommy: Baby, you have to understand that if you keep eating the way you have been, your body will keep gaining weight.

Alina: But I don't eat pizza every day.

Mommy: Yes, that's true, but I think you probably eat too much food overall, and especially fruit and sweets.

Alina: But I only eat four or five fruits a day!

Mommy: But most people eat only one or two, sweetheart. Listen, when I was graduating from high school, my acting teacher sat me down on graduation day and said to me, "Listen, Susan, you have a choice. You can either lose weight, be versatile, and have lots of different parts. Or you can stay heavy, and you will still get parts because you are talented, but you will only get certain parts that you can fit as a person who is heavy." Well, I hated her for saying that.

Alina: Why?

Mommy: Because it just seemed so mean, as if she was telling me I was fat. So I tried to forget what she said, and I didn't change. And then I found my program three years later, and things got much better.

Alina: But I'm too young for your program.

Mommy: Yes, you are. So I think the best thing to do is just relax, and don't worry about it. Don't worry.

Alina: But I hate carrying this weight.

Mommy: I know, sweetheart. I can help you if you want to change your food.

Alina [softly]: But Mommy, I can't diet. I can't.

Mommy: I understand. Neither could I. Diets make you miserable. You just feel like you want food more than ever, and you feel deprived all the time. And everyone else around you is eating everything you want!

Alina: [nodding, eyes wide]

Mommy: No, diets don't work for people like you and me. So maybe just relax, and don't worry about it right now.

Alina: Okay.

Mommy: And tomorrow Ben will be on his overnight, and Daddy's in Boston, so it can be a Mommy and Alina night!

Alina: Yay!

Mommy: Yay!

It was a good talk and, I imagine, not the last we will have on this topic. I hope I helped her feel better about herself. I think I did. But the truth is, and anyone who has lived a while and had meaningful connections with others knows, no one escapes. Life is an equal-opportunity abuser, and Alina will take her lumps.

Yet she is strong. She has had a lifetime of a brother with special needs, and yet she has maintained an unstoppable *joie de vivre* and remains a true force of nature. Notably, this issue with food and her body has nothing to do with Ben. She is her own person, with her own struggles. She is not merely a reflection of Ben's issues.

She and I are so similar. My food and weight problems transcended my brother's heart problems and handicaps. When he died, food addiction became my anesthesia. But there's hope for Alina. She's not numb. She is just a foodie with a bad metabolism and a complicated, precocious, and passionate spirit.

At least I got to be a good mom tonight. Alina is sleeping well and feeling, I think, secure and loved. That's a lot; it's enough for tonight.

OURSELVES

How does one survive it?

I survived autism by cultivating several fundamental attitudes:

- My best is enough.
- I matter, too.
- I can love, accept, and celebrate my child, *now*.

It took me years to attain these attitudes, and I maintain them imperfectly, even today. But they are my foundation, and when I practice them, I maintain my ability to face our challenges with courage and grace. *When* I practice them.

Autism challenged my immature understanding of love. I thought love was a feeling, and when Ben loved me, I would be fulfilled and happy. But it was only when I surrendered to the fact that Ben's way of loving me did not resemble at all what I thought his love would look like, that I actually connected with him in a loving relationship. Ultimately, I learned that the fulfillment of love is in the *loving*, not in the *being loved*. To plagiarize St. Francis, it's in the giving, not the getting, that one experiences love. Meeting Ben on his terms, in an act of love, gave me the experience of love. To experience an authentic relationship with my son, I had to surrender who I wanted him to be and accept who he actually was. I had to embrace the fall of my hopes to truly embrace the child standing in front of me.

SUNDAY, FEBRUARY 28, 2010

Embracing the fall

Two days ago, we had a birthday party for Alina, who turned five three days ago. Twelve five-year-olds gathered at a gymnastics studio near our house. At one point, my husband corralled all the mommies into the gym to jump into "the pit," a high jump off a wooden plank into a pool of foam. I wanted to be a team player, doing the cool thing with all the other moms, so I was the second to go, right after a friend of mine, who made it look easy.

Up I went, onto the plank, and suddenly, there I was, high, very high, above the pit, and absolutely terrified. It had looked so easy from the ground! I looked down at my husband, my daughter, the other mothers, and their children, who were all looking at me. I imagined they were wondering why I was taking so long to jump.

I think I had a mild stroke.

But I couldn't not jump; I couldn't let Alina down. So I put one foot out in front of me and then the other and then I was falling, my heart up in my throat and my lungs gasping for air because I was holding my breath, puffing out my cheeks like Dizzy Gillespie and staying scared the whole long (short) way down. I landed easily, and Alina ran over to help me crawl out.

So I did it. I jumped. I didn't let anyone down. But I did not enjoy the experience. I resisted it, and I felt my resistance deeply. I held my breath. I did not experience the moment. Afterward, that night, I thought about the experience I chose to have. I knew I was going to jump. I wanted to be "that kind of mom." But I wasn't really that kind of mom, because I didn't have fun. "That kind of mom" actually likes the experience. I was a fake "that kind of mom," and I knew it.

I thought, that night, about the symbolism for me of that moment, of doing it—sure, yeah, good job, and yay for me—but that I resisted it, so I didn't enjoy it. I do not want my life to be that way. I thought about being in the playroom with Ben. I thought about playing with Alina. I thought about all the experiences where I am "supposed" to be enjoying myself, but I'm really not because I'm scared, and I'm resisting the experience rather than surrendering and embracing it.

Truthfully, in my life, sometimes I do let go and embrace the fall, and sometimes I don't, and the difference is between living and resisting life, between living and a self-made purgatory. Life is what is happening now. Resistance and fight equal missed opportunities. When I jumped off the plank at the party, that was life, that moment was my life. And I resisted. And I stopped breathing to resist it, to not feel it. I chose fear.

I have a lot of experiences in my life where I have this choice, to embrace or resist. Going back to the gymnastics studio to jump again might not be my first choice for a free moment, but I want to embrace the fall elsewhere in my life. Embrace the opportunities. Surrender and dive in 100 percent—1000 percent! This is it. This is it right now.

So I have a choice. I can choose not to be present. I can avoid. We can go places, check out with electronics, or overschedule. I can stay busy. Or, I can be courageous and grab onto the experience of my beautiful children in their world. I can be with my children when they struggle with their different challenges. I can experiment with play and surrender my comfort. Whether I am ready, good enough, perfect enough, or not—I can show up as their mother and embrace the fall.

I still lose it, sometimes, and even that's okay. Ultimately, finally, I continue to learn how to love: my husband, both of my children, and myself.

***

The most important lesson I have learned, in surviving the autism journey, is that I will fail. I will fail at being loving. I will fail at acceptance. I will fail at taking care of myself. I will fail at being disciplined. I will fail, and fail, and fail. Yet I will continue to show up and give it my all. Even if some days my "all" stinks. I will continue to try.

Eventually, I will progress, and life—with or without autism—will continue to improve.

SUNDAY, AUGUST 17, 2014

Still angry, after all these years

Today I was packing. We are moving in three days to our new and beautiful home, five minutes away from the rental home where we have lived for the past two years. As I went through boxes of photographs, memories arose. Pictures of Ben as an infant, struggling to swallow a drop of milk through his tiny, preemie lips. Pictures of my parents holding Ben, full of joy. I remembered the years of fertility treatments, our daily hopes and prayers. I remembered our ecstasy upon finally, amazingly, finding out I was pregnant. I remember the euphoria, the passion, the indescribable ecstasy of holding my tiny son in my arms. We had hope. We had great expectations.

But then everything went wrong. What was going on? What was wrong with our son? Confusion and fear. Then the autism diagnosis, and our dreams down the toilet. Grieving our vision for our family and for our life.

I know we're not alone. I know millions of parents today are facing autism. But in certain moments, knowing that doesn't make it any better. I don't understand why my beautiful, brilliant, handsome, loving, joyful child should be so limited. I don't understand.

These feelings overtook me, and I cried. I called to Sean. He came, I told him what I was feeling, and I cried more. He held me and told me he understood, that he identified with my rage and my sadness. No matter how far along we get, there is sometimes a primal—what? Anger? Self-pity? Rage? Grief?

After some time, I returned to acceptance, and then to love. My child has to suffer. Whose child doesn't? It's okay. We continue on.

My rage is a barrier between me and Ben, so I can't allow it in. I don't want to hate his autism, or any part of him. I don't want to hate, period.

So many years in, and these feelings still come up.

WEDNESDAY, AUGUST 27, 2014

There is no ending to this story. Currently, Ben is in the throes of massive OCD. It makes sense, as he has had no structure for almost a month since camp ended. Thankfully school will resume in a week or so.

Perhaps we will return to IVIG, perhaps to CD, perhaps I will focus on diet more, and see what that does. We are seeing yet another doctor, who has diagnosed Ben with eighteen different environmental allergies, so Ben is now taking a serum for them. I'm not sure I see any changes yet.

My life continues. Sean and I continue. The family continues, and we take the moments. We sit on our deck, hold hands, and say the Serenity Prayer together, as a family. We eat our homemade, obnoxiously healthy dinner and relax. We make each other laugh. We have a family. We have a home. Sean has a good job, and I have a burgeoning career. The children love their schools. They struggle in their respective ways, but are smart, loving, and happy.

We are truly, truly blessed. It has become, incredibly, a good life.

***

PART IV:

CONCLUSION

Chapter 7
Lessons Learned

Through our years of work with Ben, we gleaned certain key points, which are summarized below. Please note that this list is not a magic bullet or a treatment roadmap, but rather a collection of internal attitudes we addressed in order to prepare ourselves to strategize for Ben's recovery.

Lesson 1. Believe in your child.
The most important lesson that we learned, and continue to learn, is to believe in Ben's potential for recovery. Regardless of what doctors, family members, and well-meaning friends may tell you, your child has the potential for connection—with you, your family members, peers, and the world around him. Believe in his potential. Believe he can heal.

Lesson 2. No one else can help your child the way you can.
Who is the greatest healer for my child? *I am.* Who is my child's greatest expert? *I am.* Whether you are the parent, grandparent, or the primary caregiver through some other circumstances, if you believe in your child's potential, and he is in your care, *you* are the one who can help him recover.

Lesson 3. You don't have to be perfect to help your child.

It is startling to realize that over six years has gone by since we began our journey of recovery with Ben. One of the most important things I learned along the way is the necessity of allowing myself to be human. As we walked the path, I fell apart sometimes, threw temper tantrums, and had self-pity binges. My husband and I often struggled to remain hopeful in the face of setbacks and the intermittent resumption of Ben's autistic symptoms. We did nothing perfectly, but we have gone along willingly and persistently. Our consistent actions and love for our child, rather than our inevitably complicated feelings, were what mattered.

If I can help Ben get well, then I believe any mother, father, or caregiver who wants recovery for his or her child badly enough can do it, too. And how do I define "get well"? Cure? *Maybe.* Improvement and progress? *Definitely.* Connection and a more meaningful relationship with your child? *Absolutely.* We don't need to be perfect parents with perfect skills, and we don't need perfect children. This process is about the perfection of love as a driving force to motivate us on a challenging and enlightening journey of connection with our children.

I hated autism. I wanted my son. Today, I don't hate autism, but I also don't want my son and family to suffer from it. Today, we don't have to. When I look at who Ben is today—a functioning, happy, interactive, expressive, deeply-connected child—and compare him to who he was when we began our journey—a child totally imprisoned in autism—I realize that somehow, I have been, done, and loved him enough.

Lesson 4. Cultivate certain internal practices.

In order for Ben to grow, *we* needed to do the following:

- Fall in love with every part of Ben, *including his autism*—this took a long time, for both my husband and me.

- Learn to accept, be with, and celebrate our child *now*—*before* he acquires the skills we hoped he would someday.
- Learn to *study* our child: observe, take notes, and make note of his responses to every intervention we tried. This was a skill I had to develop. I tend to be a big-picture person; I had to learn to pay attention to the details, so that I wouldn't miss subtle pieces of information about Ben's condition at any given moment.

Lesson 5. Ask the right questions.

After years of exploration, research, and ultimately successful intervention, we realized Ben's process came down to several key questions:

A. *What inspires your child?* When you discover your child's motivations, you discover a bridge across the chasm of disconnection, the chasm that is, of course, the hallmark of autism. Our initial step with Ben was to connect with him *on his terms,* through the discovery, based on close observation, of what motivated him. This was a core Son-Rise Program principle. As Ben realized that we wanted to play *his* games, on *his* terms, and have fun in *his* way, a pivotal change occurred: *he became invested.* He started to want a relationship with us. Once Ben wanted to connect with us, his brain found a way to rewrite the neural pathways and make that connection happen. Without that pivotal step of igniting Ben's own desire for connection, the chasm of disconnection would have remained uncrossable, regardless of any biomedical interventions.

B. *What does your child receive from his environment in the form of food, and how well is his digestive system able to process the food he takes in?* In other words, how successfully does your child's digestive system extract and process nutrients that are critical to his internal systems?

C. *What does your child receive from his or her environment in the form of toxins (e.g., chemicals, electromagnetic radiation, heavy metals), and how well can his or her immune system purge such toxins?* In other words, to what degree does your child's body contain harmful toxins (*e.g.*, parasites, colonic backup, a clogged liver, or other poisons) that prevent the healthy functioning of his or her internal systems, including your child's neurological and immune systems?

D. *Do you truly want to pursue this path?* In our experience, this path is frightening to many parents. The idea that your child can make meaningful progress, and possibly even recover, but that you yourselves have to play a part in that recovery, is terrifying. These were some of the questions with which I plagued myself over the years of our journey:

    a. What if I am inadequate, and my child's failure to heal is my fault?

    b. What if we can't afford the financial costs?

    c. What if my partner and I both have to work and don't have sufficient time to invest in our child's recovery?

    d. What about our other child who also needs our attention and care?

    e. How on earth will I be able to handle what feels like a completely overwhelming set of steps to take?

    f. What if I try this path, and my child doesn't get better? What does that say about *me*?

Indeed, there is something to be said for running like hell in the opposite direction once you have read this book and heard what we endured. But once we were able to discern the *right questions,* we were on our way to finding the *right answers* to vastly improving Ben's condition and our own situation.

Lesson 6. Find the right answers for your *child.*
The answers to *your* child's autism will be unique to your child. Many interventions that worked for other families did not work for Ben. Conversely, many methods that helped Ben have gotten other children nowhere. In sum, our answers to Ben's autism so far have been (a) his Son-Rise Program, through which he was nurtured, supported, and ultimately inspired to desire connection with others; (b) nutritional interventions, through which his digestive system became able to function more effectively; (c) detoxification and supplementation, through which his immune system became able to respond effectively to toxicity in his body, purging him of harmful organisms that interfere with proper brain function; and (d) supportive counseling and lifestyle training for us as parents, through which we found the hope and strength to love our child and follow this path to its present, much-improved point.

These were *our* answers, for *our* child, and for *our* family. The path offers no guarantees, and your child's unique constitution, genetic predisposition, and family history will determine his or her needs and solutions.

Become a private detective. Your child, your life with your child, and the life of your family—they're worth it.

Lesson 7. Accept the ups and downs. They have lessons to teach you.
The greatest challenge for me, throughout the journey, and to this day remains the unpredictability of the process. Often, Ben seemed to be doing well, and then suddenly, without any apparent explanation, he would exhibit autistic symptoms again. Ultimately, I learned enough about Ben's autism, its causes and triggers, to understand why these

symptoms recurred. For Ben, the root always seems to be an organic problem, such as a yeast reaction to an excess of a certain type of food or a hormonal imbalance brought on by poor sleep.

In addition, Ben is also acutely emotionally sensitive. Time after time, as he learned rudimentary social skills, he stumbled badly, like a toddler learning to walk, and experienced rejection from his peers. These experiences devastated him emotionally, and we usually saw autistic symptoms almost immediately afterwards. Ben's emotional life strongly influences his immune system, so that when he is hit emotionally, he is hit immunologically as well. His impaired immune system in turn impedes his neural functioning, and autistic symptoms return.

Today it is much easier for me to accept the ebb and flow of his behaviors, even if they are troubling. It's easier for two reasons: first, because the swings up and down are much less dramatic and second, because I know he will detox himself sooner or later and resolve whatever issues he is processing, either emotionally or organically.

Lesson 8. Take care of your own needs, and parent yourself as you would parent your child.

I learned that my capacity to accept and flow with Ben's changes are directly proportional to my degree of *self-care*. If I neglect myself—exercise, sleep, emotional support, and so forth—Ben's social challenges wreck me. But if I remember that self-caring is not the same as selfishness, and prioritize my own needs as well as Ben's, I have much more emotional Teflon against his fluctuations.

Finally, and most importantly, I learned to love myself unconditionally and forgive myself for being a human being and a mother, rather than a healer or a god. I became able to love without expectation.

For whatever reason, I had to learn this lesson with Ben first, and *then* apply that lesson to myself.

FINAL THOUGHTS

The autism statistics are staggering, even inconceivable. Every day, more families are affected. Sadly, most of them at this point in time have no idea of the resources immediately available to help their children and themselves. Still, there is hope. Growing numbers of families are banding together to support one another as we endeavor to heal our children. In-person and online support groups abound for families experiencing autism. Practitioners, even allopathic, Western doctors, are starting to open their minds to the concept of *autism recovery*.

The autism recovery journey is costly in every conceivable way. But so is a lifetime of managed care for a person with autism. I'd rather do my hard work now and try for a better future for all of us, than have our family consigned to lives enslaved by autism. Ben is a vision of hope for any family suffering with autism. That hope, more than anything, is why I wrote this book. I'm grateful we took this road. I hope this book will inspire you to take it, too.

In the end, autism turned out to be a vehicle for intense emotional and personal growth for my husband and me. It took a long time, and a lot of good moments, to heal the emotional wounds left by our early experiences. But through our experience with Ben's autism, we learned to love our child unconditionally, and for that I will always be grateful. We learned to love Ben without needing him to be someone he wasn't and without expectations. I learned to love the child who *was* in front of me and to be deeply and truly grateful for who he was—and is. Learning to love Ben in this way ultimately taught me to love the other people in my life, especially my husband and my daughter, in a totally different way. I came to see them as they are, without judgment, rather than comparing them to some vision of the people I want them to be.

This road is hard. But it's worth it.

I used to think my son didn't see me. Today, I know my son *always* saw me. He just didn't know how to show it.

I used to think my son didn't love me. Today, I know my son *always* loved me. He just didn't have the tools to express it.

Whatever you choose for your child's treatment, know that your child loves you—whether he can show it today or not.

Epilogue

A wonderful start

Today was the first day of Ben's third year at Otto Specht, and as always, it began with an assembly. Remarkably, the assembly room was filled with the families of new students. Some of the parents even gasped as they entered the hall. We all commented happily on the school's growth since the past year.

The families sat patiently, waiting for the children to appear. All of a sudden, the school's accompanist began to play "The Minstrel Boy," a tune that always heralds the entrance of the children. Sure enough, the children began to file in slowly, grinning and elegant, dressed in their assembly clothing. I saw Ben, catalogue-handsome in his white Oxford shirt and blue blazer, new blue braces shining out. The students seated themselves in the two front rows of the hall.

During the assembly, the school's director led us through an hour-long experience of music, intermixed with introductions and story telling. A high-school student, new to the school, sat in the second row. Frequently during the assembly, he spoke out freely, asking questions and making loud comments at inappropriate moments. He was enthusiastic and charming, though clearly unaware of the rules of assembly etiquette. His parents, new friends of mine, sat nearby, smiling. I wondered what they were feeling.

Suddenly, my mind shot back to two years earlier, September 10, 2012, our own first assembly at Otto Specht. Sean and I sat together that morning, our palms sweating, as Ben shot out comments, interrupted with charming, enthusiastic, but ill-timed questions, got up at one point to dance a little jig, and had absolutely no sense of the inappropriateness of his actions.

Today, that Ben was gone. The Ben at this morning's assembly sat quietly, patiently, and happily throughout the assembly, sang his favorite songs with obvious pleasure, and filed in and out of the hall without incident. At one point he even graced me with a grin and a wave. After the assembly, however, I became "uncool Mom," and Ben disappeared immediately into his day, without even a hello. No problem, my darling!

Later in the day, I ran into two of Ben's teachers, both of whom have known Ben since he started at Otto Specht. Both of them burst out with celebrations of Ben's maturity and transformation since that first assembly. The contrast was radical. We *kvelled* for a bit and then it was time to go pick up Alina.

Our new school year had begun.

Afterword

A Conversation with Donna Gates on Autism Prevention through Lifestyle Choices

Donna Gates is an internationally renowned nutritionist and author of The Body Ecology Diet. *Donna works extensively with children with autism as well as adults with numerous health issues. I consulted with Donna several times over the past few years for help with Ben's diet and supplement regimen. While speaking with me recently about this book, Donna exclaimed, "You have to have a chapter on autism prevention, so parents know what to do!" Since our story effectively begins with diagnosis, rather than prevention, I asked Donna if I could interview her for the chapter. That interview follows below. For more about Donna, go to www.bodyecology.com.*

Where does autism come from?

Today we find ourselves at the heart of a perfect storm. We have a generation of children coming in right now who are showing us that what we've been doing for the last four or five generations has been wrong in terms of the ways in which we have been feeding our bodies and all the toxins that we're dumping into them. This generation is paying the price.

Today we're seeing children that look good on the outside, but who are nutritionally depleted. Their parents haven't eaten well, have a lot of toxins in their bodies, and are passing those toxins on from generation to generation. In the early 1900s, we started altering our diet considerably. It got worse with the baby boomers, many of whom ate TV dinners on aluminum trays and ate lots of sugar and fructose. To this day, people are unconscious; in other words, they don't realize that when you put unhealthy foods into your body, you're going to pay for it. That's what's happening today: we are paying for it and so are our children.

Children today are born with a lot of inflammation because we have a serious epidemic of candidiasis, resulting from an overuse of antibiotics, among other things. Today, women have yeast infections to varying degrees, of which they might not be aware. When they enter pregnancy, that yeast infection becomes much more acute. During pregnancy, the mother's progesterone, estrogen, and glucose levels all increase, which is healthy for the pregnancy, but can also lead to candidiasis. As a result, many babies today are born with a yeast infection. I have in fact never worked with a child with autism who didn't have, as an infant, symptoms of candidiasis, such as cradle cap, skin rashes, diaper rashes, and so on; digestive disorders; or thrush in their mouth. Candidiasis is a systemic infection that mothers unknowingly pass on to their babies. But if these women become aware that their children are going to be born with a yeast infection, before the baby is conceived, they can start doing things to help throw that infection off.

Is autism genetic?

Today, many genes are showing up indicating a predisposition to autism. Many children that don't have autism, however, also have those same genetic variations, and I don't think it's a genetic cause *per se*. We have to look at the microbes in our gut and the profound effect they have on the immune system. That being said, we do need to look at genes, especially whether these particular kids are poor detoxifiers and whether the mother and the father are as well. If so, they're likely to pass that on to their child. So it's very important that both parents are tested.

How do you decrease the likelihood of autism?

First of all, you don't want to wait until the baby comes into the world to start. I recommend that both of the potential parents do at least a six-month detox program prior to conception and get tested for heavy metals. They may even want to do an aggressive detox program where they're doing colonics and using supplements or chelation to get heavy metals and other toxins out of their body.

At the very least, they should be on a diet that's more of what people today are calling a Paleo diet. We at Body Ecology have had a Paleo diet for twenty years, though we didn't call it that. Body Ecology is a gluten-free diet that is also sugar-free. What sets Body Ecology apart is that we also encourage people to eat fermented foods, that is, probiotic foods. Parents planning to conceive should spend at least six months on this diet prior to conception.

One of the beautiful things about autism is that people are now realizing we have to take better care of our kids, and that we have to take better care of mothers during pregnancy. What happens during the pregnancy is terribly important, because although the baby has a set of genes that are clearly defined and formed, throughout the entire pregnancy, the mother's lifestyle choices affect the expression of those genes. So if during her pregnancy the mother is eating well and she's at peace, her baby has a greater chance of being healthy and happy. What happens in the womb determines the longevity and health of the child throughout its entire life. Family members should, therefore, pamper the mother to help ensure that her pregnancy is happy, healthy, and relaxed, and that she sleeps well and has as little stress as possible. Everybody should participate in the development of that child.

What about a mom who is, for example, working two jobs, is pregnant, and doesn't have support? What would you recommend for someone like that?

She had a partner. If that partner is no longer present, the mother needs to feed herself well by having simple meals of high-quality foods. She also needs to realize that how she perceives the stress she's under determines its impact on her. The more she connects with her child and sends wonderful, happy thoughts to him or her, the less impact the stress in her life will have on her baby.

What are some of the most important actions a mother can take with respect to diet before and during pregnancy?

The use of fermented foods is terribly important because they're rich in healthy bacteria that put good bacteria in the gut. Those bacteria help to keep the mother's cells clean so the baby that's forming will have less toxins as it develops. Vegetables, for example, are very rich in antioxidants; greens especially are powerful cleansers. Fermenting cruciferous vegetables—already powerful cleansers for the body—maximizes their cleansing effect.

If the mother eats fermented vegetables with at least two meals a day, then she provides better nutrition to her child, because fermenting vegetables also increases the bioavailability of the vegetable's nutrients. Cabbage, for example, is rich in Vitamin C, but the Vitamin C is hundreds of times more bioavailable in fermented cabbage (sauerkraut). Furthermore, when you eat probiotic foods with other foods, the probiotic microbes help break down and digest the other foods as well, providing far superior nutrition.

Kefir is also great to drink before, during, and after pregnancy because it's an extremely powerful cleanser for the liver, heart, and blood. Women tend to get constipated during pregnancy, when progesterone increases. Progesterone actually slows down the movement of food through the digestive tract. It's nature's fail-safe mechanism in pregnancy to ensure that the food doesn't move through the mother's body so fast that the baby can't be nourished. But it's very important that during pregnancy a mother not let herself get constipated, so I recommend lower-bowel enemas—which are completely safe during pregnancy—if the mother becomes constipated.

I also recommend protein twice a day, around 11:00 and 1:30, two small, protein meals. Eggs are excellent, because they are rich in DHA, which is great for the baby's brain. In some countries, like China, a woman will eat ten eggs a day if she is pregnant. Ideally, the eggs will be fertile eggs, because they have been shown to be more digestible.

Women today worry about fish during pregnancy. But if you have a piece of fish with fermented vegetables, the beneficial bacteria in the vegetables will eat up the toxins, because one of their jobs is to clean up their environment and keep parasites and eggs from forming. In sum, I recommend protein, cultured vegetables, dark-green, leafy vegetables, vegetables from the cruciferous family, and ocean vegetables, which provide a great source of minerals.

Sugar, chocolate, and coffee should be avoided during pregnancy, because they can be extremely stimulating for the baby, who may in fact have a genetic variation whereby he or she can't clear those substances and may become hyperactive. Moreover, a vegetarian mother who's eating a lot of greens, legumes, nuts, seeds, and so on can absorb too much copper from those foods and then must take more zinc. A diet that's rich in copper-based foods can cause copper overload, which can do harm to the baby's brain. Typically, we need animal protein because it provides zinc, so if a mother eats a vegetarian diet, she's got to supplement her zinc. The book, *Why Am I So Tired*, by Ann Louise Gittleman, does a great job of explaining this copper–zinc imbalance and the damage that can occur to the mother's and baby's brains from the fatigue that results from that imbalance. Women should have their nutrients tested before they get pregnant to determine both their zinc and copper status.

What do you think about exercise during pregnancy?
The body needs energy to grow a child, and exercising too aggressively uses up a lot of energy. In Asian countries, for example, they would frown on a woman who became pregnant, had an extremely active lifestyle, and didn't choose to slow down that lifestyle during her pregnancy. But in America, pregnant women get on airplanes and travel and keep on going in so many ways, and in so doing deplete their bodies of the energy needed for their baby's healthy development. Calming forms of exercise, like walking and yoga, are safe to do and should be done. Walking, for example, helps women with constipation because of the hip movement. Swimming, though relaxing for some people, can be problematic in pregnancy because of chlorinated pool water.

Do you see a relationship between GMO foods and autism?
I don't. The harmful effect of genetically modified foods on the gut is substantial, but I don't think that that's the cause of autism. Fundamentally, the gut of the mother while she's carrying the baby needs to be healthy, and then after birth, the baby needs to be supported to develop and maintain a healthy gut. Again, eating fermented foods is protective, because you are constantly putting in healthy new bacteria that are going to control the environment because there's so many of them because you're always eating them. That's the protection against genetically modified foods.

It's certainly important to avoid genetically modified foods, but you don't necessarily need to buy all organic foods. The critical issue is whether the produce has been sprayed. Some nonorganic farmers are actually better than the organic ones, because they don't spray.

They aren't certified, but their produce is actually better than the ones that are so-called "certified organic." So even if you aren't able to buy organic or unsprayed vegetables, eat the plant foods anyway, because they are so important.

Fermented vegetables will protect you. In Body Ecology, we recommend protein in your meals, but 80 percent of your plate should be vegetables. Fermented vegetables are the protective mechanism that is going to help us get through this period of time where so much of our food is, in fact, genetically modified and poisoned.

How much fermented food should we eat at our meals?

Two to three tablespoons of fermented (cultured) vegetables at each meal is ideal, and for pregnant women, eight ounces a day of coconut kefir. You can also buy probiotic liquids, and just a couple of ounces of those two or three times a day, or with a meal, will be wonderfully helpful. I do not recommend Kombucha because of the wild yeast. Wild fermentation increases the amount of yeast you are ingesting. Apple cider vinegar produces acetic acid, which is beneficial, rather than lactic acid, which is harmful. Apple cider vinegar is actually a medicinal form of fermentation.

How would a woman who is planning a pregnancy, or currently pregnant, make her way through the aisles and aisles of supplements, protein powders, fish oils, and everything else available on the market? Which products are essential?

Since the brain needs DHA, I recommend taking a fish-oil supplement that's high in DHA. Krill oil, which is assimilated easily into the brain, is also an excellent choice. Additionally, women need to increase their intake of fresh, pastured butter when they are pregnant, because 50 percent of the energy that comes from breast milk going to the baby is in the fat in the milk. The butter will increase the fat content in breast milk, as well as increase milk production overall.

In pregnancy, our nutritional needs change, so many women who can't tolerate milk normally find they can actually do very well on it during pregnancy, especially if they choose fermented goat's milk or other A2 casein-based milks. Cow's milk is A1 casein, which is much harder for humans to digest.

What kind of water should women drink before and during pregnancy?
I don't think anyone should trust their city-water systems, because they are too old and outdated, and the cities don't have the money to bring them up to par. Ideally, people should have their water tested before pregnancy, but certainly during the pregnancy and while a mother is breast-feeding, to ensure that they have the cleanest water possible.

Reverse osmosis produces clean water, but it needs minerals added to it. Adding fulvic minerals to your water is tremendously beneficial. You can buy liquid fulvic minerals and use half a drop in a glass of water or a dropper in a big bottle of water that you can drink throughout the day. You can also have one or two glasses of water a day with a quarter of a teaspoon of Celtic sea salt added to it, which will support the adrenals.

Once again, you may not always be aware that the things you are eating and drinking have toxins in them. So the fermented vegetables and kefirs will be your fail-safe mechanisms, because they scavenge for toxins and will keep your gut healthy.

Do you have any other suggestions regarding helping a child with autism?
Do not instill in the mind of your child that he is autistic or that he has been labeled as having something wrong with him. That belief

buried in his subconscious mind, even from the earliest stages of life, can create a huge barrier to healing for him. So much of what we create in our lives is from what we believe in our subconscious minds, and mothers have a tremendous influence on their children through their words and actions. Even fetuses have a sensing brain, so if the mother's worried or upset or happy and joyful, the baby is already sensing her feelings and emotions. And they never lose that connection.

So it's important to have a positive attitude around your child. If you believe your child is going to get well, they'll believe they're going to get well, too—and then their chances of getting well will increase. There was one mother I spoke with who never told her autistic son that he had anything wrong with him. They just told him he had problems with his tummy. They didn't let him know there was anything seriously wrong with him; they actually made it clear that there *wasn't* anything wrong with him. He's extremely healthy and normal today. He has no memory whatsoever of being unwell. He had autism, but he doesn't know that he did.

The other side is that the parents also label themselves. They begin to define themselves as "the parents of an autistic child." Whether it's motivated by a desire for status and sympathy, the label ultimately comes to define them and comprise their self-definition in a negative way. There are professionals who work with parents on these issues, people like Darren Weitzman and Roxanne Bachman, and Carl Dawson over in England. These kind of therapies need to be brought in.

I agree strongly. Every parent I talk to who has a child on the spectrum seems to carry a huge burden of guilt, as well as deep-seated feelings of unworthiness. They believe they have failed their children. This autism epidemic is happening to parents as well as to the children.

Finally, is there anything that you can suggest regarding how to prepare oneself and one's children, especially if you have a picky eater, for entering this new world of understanding and respecting the connection between food and your baby's health? How does one avoid getting total overwhelmed?

In Body Ecology, we focus on universal principles, which enable us to tackle this enormous challenge of living a healthy life in an unhealthy world. One of the most important is the principle of *step-by-step*. Like a universe, learning to eat and live healthfully advances forward in tiny increments. We age in tiny increments. Day comes on in tiny increments, and night comes on in tiny increments. We have to follow that order. You can't do too much too fast, or you'll fail.

You begin with the things that are going to create the most energy. Specifically, you need to focus on your thyroid and adrenal glands, and on getting enough sleep. In this country, our lifestyle habits are so unhealthy. Moms in particular. For example, when we finally get some time to ourselves, instead of getting ourselves into bed or something, we stay up and answer e-mails or watch a TV show. And the show might be exciting and raise our cortisol levels, so we don't sleep well that night. It's important to pamper yourself and get a good night's sleep, to truly take care of ourselves.

We also focus on conquering infections. Change your diet to eliminate the unhealthy sugars and add in fermented foods. Change the diet, add fermented foods, get more rest, and the energy will change tremendously. If the mother's healthier, stronger, and feeling better, she's going to do a better job of taking care of herself and her family. Also, because part of the principle is also to cleanse out toxins, I recommend home enemas for any child with autism, because they eliminate the toxins so quickly.

Finally, you correct digestion by preparing the food so it's easy to digest, and also using enzymes. If your child is old enough, he or she can swallow capsules; otherwise, you can put plant enzymes in his or her food and stir it in to help digestion.

So, once again, where do you start?

At the very beginning, if you were to make just one change, take one first step, it should be to add the fermented foods. They change the gut, which changes the brain. For the mothers to change their children's diets, they need to start with their own diets first. If they improve their own diets, it will be much easier to turn around and hand it to their children. You start eating the new foods. Your child sees you eating them. You then turn around and serve them to your child.

Rather than feeling guilty for focusing on yourself, cultivate the belief that if you help yourself first, it will be easier to help your child.

Acknowledgments

This book is the result of the service and love our family received over the past seven years from countless people who assisted us mentally, spiritually, emotionally, and logistically.

In particular, there are several groupings of people to whom I am grateful:

Alina, my ebullient burst of primary colors and my mirror; Ben, my endlessly unfolding and blossoming boy; Sean, my partner in all the things that matter; my parents, who give me love, joy, wisdom, and perspective; Bears and Samahria Kaufman, "Captain William" and Bryn Hogan, Becky and Carolina; all of our Son-Rise "homeschool teachers," including but not limited to Julie Hudson and Leah Hughes, Kermit Chavez and Herzon Gutierrez, Steve Alves, Sana Semeniuk, Oscar Gui, our beloved North Watt, Chelsea Stewart, Jake Cawley, German Jessy, Justine Waldron, Katie Mellman, Carla Recinos, Meegan Alves, Florian Kessler, Hendrik Diefenbach, Dylan Ripke-Thorne, and many others who gave their time and love to Ben and to us; Tony Lyons and Skyhorse Press; my editor, Jonathan Arlan, the most affable editor I've ever met; all of my advance readers; my beloved mother-in-law, Grandma Ro; Jonathan Alderson, who advised me skillfully and compassionately at a very rough time; Mary Holland, without whom this book would not have happened; Amanda Mecke, my stalwart guide and agent; Milly Marmur, my literary godmother; Nancy O'Hara, M.D. and Gail Szakacs, M.D., who brought Ben seven leagues forward; Donna Gates, who helps so many; Tim Miller, my stalwart source of sarcasm and silliness; Jeanette Rodriguez, whose vision for Otto Specht gave my child a place to be; everyone who read my blog and commented or encouraged me; Claudine Kaplan, my Waldorf-inspired guiding light; Bill and Bob and Cynthia, who collectively taught me how to live like a grown-up; Carol Castle, Diane O'Keeffe, Lynne Skinner, David Irvine, George Masselam, and Christine Williams, through whom God often works to hold me together; and finally, Jamie Myers and Kat Crawford, who love all of us so much and gave me two of the most beautiful workspaces any writer could ever ask for to complete the first draft.

Most important, thanks to God, and to the other parents who love their children and are working to help them heal.

Connect With Susan

After years of learning how to help my family "unlock" our potential for healing and happiness, I am now passionate about helping other families do the same. Every family's goal is health and happiness, but most of us need help to reach that destination.

At my website, www.RoadsToFamilyWellness.com, you can access:

- Information about my family health coaching programs;
- Referrals to practitioners I trust and programs I believe in for treating autism, ADHD, and other prevalent childhood disorders;
- Updates on the Levin family's ongoing journey; and,
- Free downloads of Ben's short stories for children.

You can also sign up for my newsletter, which will keep you abreast of my ongoing research into new interventions, additional sources of support, and my latest recipes.

I hope this book has given you, or someone you love, hope for your family's brighter future.